Advance Praise for *The Pain-Free Program*

"For decades orthopedists and neurosurgeons told me I'd simply have to put up with my bad back. Anthony Carey told me otherwise. I've been living pain free ever since."

—Parvez Mahmood, M.D., F.A.C.S.

"We all have the capacity to make positive changes to how our body functions and feels. Anthony's book will walk you through the simple steps of seeing where help is needed and what you can do about it. It's your body—and, for the most part—you are in charge."

—Morrissey, Multiplatinum recording artist and former lead singer of the Smiths

"Years of triathlon training and countless international airline flights take a toll on your body in their own unique way. The philosophy that Anthony Carey promotes and practices can erase years of misuse."

—Jeff Jacobs, President of Global Development for Qualcomm

"*The Pain-Free Program* is a practical, safe, and effective approach for anyone to take control of their pain. This is a must-have book for those that want to keep control of their health, enhance their life, and live actively."

—Tom Campanaro, CEO/President of EFI Sports Medicine and Total Gym

"With this book, Anthony Carey is breaking new ground in presenting ways to help us all lead healthier lives."

—David Meggyesy, Western Director of the N.F.L. Players Association

"As a longtime dance and fitness advocate, I have always understood the importance of proper body alignment and body mechanics. Anthony Carey explains these concepts in depth and provides easy-to-follow exercises to maintain, regain, or prevent loss of physical mobility. I have sent many friends and associates to Anthony, and the result has been lots of happy, pain-free bodies."

—Judi Sheppard Missett, Jazzercise Founder and CEO

"Read this book and open your eyes to a world of possibilities and hope for helping your aches and pains."

—Greg Nelson, Cofounder and Board of Directors of Bregg Orthopedics

"*The Pain-Free Program* is not just an exercise regime, but a lifestyle that will free its followers from many physical disabilities and chronic pain. Anthony Carey's simple, yet eloquent book is the key to a pain free life. I am walking proof of that."

—Peter Kovacs, Former President and CEO of Nutrasweet

THE
PAIN-FREE
PROGRAM

A Proven Method to Relieve Back, Neck, Shoulder, and Joint Pain

ANTHONY CAREY, M.A., CSCS, CES

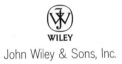

WILEY

John Wiley & Sons, Inc.

Published by John Wiley & Sons, Inc., Hoboken, New Jersey
Published simultaneously in Canada

Design and composition by Navta Associates, Inc.

Library of Congress Cataloging-in-Publication Data:

Carey, Anthony.
   The Pain-Free Program : a proven method to relieve back, neck, shoulder, and joint pain / Anthony Carey.
      p.   cm.
   ISBN-13 978-0-471-68720-7 (paper: alk. paper)
   ISBN-10 0-471-68720-0 (paper: alk. paper)
   1.   Chronic pain—Exercise therapy. I. Title.
   RB127.C375 2005
   616'.0472—dc22
                                                      2005001258

Printed in the United States of America

10 9 8 7 6 5 4 3 2 1

To Champagne, my wife and my soul mate.
If everyone could experience the kind of happiness
and love that you bring to my life,
the world would be a much better place.

Contents

Acknowledgments

First, I would like to thank the thousands of clients who have come through the doors of our office and trusted me in their time of need. I have learned something from each and every one of you. I am continually inspired by your courage, dedication, and willingness to take responsibility for your own well-being. I am a better practitioner and a better person thanks to you.

My parents, Patricia and Patrick Carey, have always been there for me with love, support, and encouragement throughout my life. The values and the ethics they raised me with have given me the necessary tools to see this project through. One of the most rewarding things in my life is to see them proud of their children.

I would also like to thank my business partner, Aaron Brooks. We came to the business as friends and will someday leave the business, still as friends. Aaron's skills as a practitioner and his integrity as a business partner have been essential to the success of our business.

I will also like to thank the members of my Mastermind Group, Harold Fox, Dennis Santopietro, and Fracka Future. Their support, motivation, and drive are an ongoing source of personal and professional growth. They have seen me along the way through the entire process.

My friend and colleague Devon Kidd volunteered her time to help me by posing for some of the exercise photos. Devon's mission is to help others (www.mentorfitness.org). Tina Luu's talent through the lens and photo editing skills were a tremendous contribution to the appearance of the book. Ze Valagao's unbelievable artistic ability and understanding of the human body brought the Categories of the bodies to life for me. My editor Teryn Johnson's patience with me through the process and her critical eye for editing have made this book something we can all be proud of. Many thanks to all of you.

Introduction

If you are in pain, all you can think about is relief. For more than twelve years, I've worked with people just like you who have endured months, years, even decades of pain that ruled their lives. Well, I'm here to tell you that it doesn't have to be that way. In this book, I've combined all of my knowledge and experience into one pain-free program that truly works. I promise that once you finish this book, not only will you have the tools you need to get rid of pain for good, you'll also possess the knowledge to keep your body healthy and functional for the rest of your life.

As far as health-care concerns go, cardiovascular issues such as heart disease and high blood pressure get most of the media's attention. While it's true that cardiovascular disease affects the *quantity* of your life, musculoskeletal problems affect the *quality* of your life. When you're in pain, you're not really living—rather, you've turned your entire focus toward managing your discomfort. Because of the pain, you're less likely to do any exercise, which can lead to those cardiovascular problems we hear so much about. In short, pain can be at the center of a vicious cycle that can undermine your happiness and your health.

If you understand that your pain is the product of many physical and environmental factors that preceded it, you can develop a strategy for change. I hope to provide a sensible guide to everyday events that are roadblocks to healing. We'll look at the body, beginning with "what" hurts, to understanding "why" it hurts. Some core concepts of my program are the interdependency of all the body's parts and the realization that a pain in one area of your body can result from other things going wrong far removed from that site of pain.

There is never a "one-size-fits-all" approach to addressing the body's aches and pains. The more individually designed an exercise program is, the more effective it will be. Books, handouts, and videos that show a group of exercises for a specific ailment deny the uniqueness of each person's body. If you and your significant other both suffer from lower-back pain, you each suffer for different reasons because your bodies are different. So, why would you do the same exercises? This book not only addresses the individuality of your physical structure, it will also let you further personalize the program by relating your exercises to the activities you do most often. If you focus on teaching the body to function correctly and stop beating itself up, you'll be rewarded with a reduction in pain.

Chronic pain has far-reaching implications for our society, even for individuals who are not in pain. Pain costs money. Pain causes lost workdays. Pain reduces productivity. Reduced productivity results in higher costs, which are eventually passed on to you—the consumer. These financial implications should matter to everyone because they affect all of us.

Function First opened its doors in 1994, empowering people to control their lives by helping them function pain-free. Our program has benefited people who felt hopeless because we looked beyond the symptoms that everyone else was chasing. Since then, we've had the good fortune of helping people from all over the United States, South America, and Europe. The Function First philosophy works because when the body is given the right stimuli (exercises), it will function and heal the way it was designed to.

If you suffer from chronic back, neck, or shoulder pain, this book will help you find lasting relief. You'll learn to assess and treat the underlying causes of your pain. Part one describes the way our bodies work. Don't skip that section because you need to understand the Function First philosophy to obtain maximum benefit. Unless you read anatomy textbooks in your spare time, you'll also appreciate the explanations of your muscles and how they function.

Part two will help you apply the Function First philosophy to your unique situation and will start you on the path toward pain relief. Find your body type and your occupation type, then go to the exercises that correspond to these. How you use your body every day makes a big difference in the type of exercises that you need to correct your pain.

If people come into our program and don't do their homework, they're fired. I can't help you if you aren't willing to do your part. So, as you read this book, keep in mind that at the end of the day, you need to put this advice into practice.

The goal of this book is not to dismiss the medical system, but to open you up to the possibility that the route you have always taken may not be the best one. If nothing else, that route is certainly not the only one. There are many ways to help yourself and your body.

Addressing the alignment of the body's structure and its relationship to how you move is based on fundamental principles of physics and the human anatomy. The relationship between posture and pain is well documented in scientific literature. By not trying to "fix" anyone's symptoms and by addressing alignment and movement, we provide the body with an opportunity to restore and heal itself.

To the millions who suffer from chronic back, neck, and shoulder pain, you can exercise the Function First way to relief in the comfort of your own home. This book will give you the essential tools and instructions to determine which Category you best fit into and what exercise program suits your lifestyle. The clear explanations and their accompanying illustrations will allow you to exercise at home without the need for expensive equipment or help from a professional. You can work at your own pace and allow your body to be your guide. You'll be in charge.

Before we get to those exercises, however, I feel that it's essential for you to thoroughly understand the human body—how it functions and how all of its parts work together. Then, it will be easy for you to see how a problem in one part of the body can relate to many other factors.

When I work privately with clients, I initially educate them about the Function First philosophy and how the process can change their lives. This is an absolute "must" before I even begin an assessment on someone. Your mind must be open to a new paradigm for achieving long-term health, and you must be able to relate that paradigm to your individual circumstances. You will be incredibly empowered by understanding the reasoning behind these exercises. If you read this book from start to finish, you'll learn that

- It's best to address the cause of pain and physical limitations, not the pain or the limitation itself.

- The body should be treated as a highly integrated structure—not as a series of unrelated parts.

- You can provide an optimal healing environment by removing daily "micro" injuries to your body.

- The Function First philosophy has a positive effect on spinal disorders and back pain, various joint pains, cumulative trauma disorders, headaches, and similar challenges.

- By addressing the cause, you are also preventing a reoccurrence of the same pain.

- It's possible to transfer the responsibility of an individual's health back to that person if you provide him or her with the tools for self-help.

You don't have to be an athlete to benefit from the Function First approach. With this program, everyone wins:

- the aging person
- the injured worker
- the accident victim
- athletes of all levels
- pain sufferers everywhere

People who win the biggest are those who can now overcome obstacles that they never knew existed. Please use these ideas and tools to take control of your own well-being for the rest of your life.

Part One

How Our Body Talks to Us

1

The Path to Pain

If you are reading this book, you are probably among the thousands of frustrated, angry people who are looking for help with their physical challenges and pain. According to the American Academy of Orthopedic Surgeons, for thirty-five million Americans—that's one in every seven—their movement is restricted by a musculoskeletal disorder, such as a broken bone, myofascial pain, arthritis, or a sports trauma. Pain sufferers are everywhere, from all walks of life and all ethnic backgrounds, socioeconomic levels, and ages. The common thread connecting these individuals is pain, either chronic (typically defined as pain that lasts longer than three months) or acute (pain that has more of a rapid onset to levels that often motivate a person to seek intervention).

Perhaps the pain you have is new. Maybe it's one more pain in a long list of pains that has prompted you to finally take action. Or maybe it's chronic pain that never went away or has disappeared, only to come back again. These scenarios often develop when chronic pain is improperly addressed over time. When this happens, the damage exceeds the body's level of tolerance, and the pain becomes acute. If intervention does not occur, disability or loss of function may result.

Maybe it's a pain that you're tired of treating with medication. The medication may not be helping any more, or perhaps its side effects have created their own problems. It could be a pain that you know is getting worse or will get worse if you don't do something about it.

You might not even experience "pain" per se, but you do have a muscular-related physical limitation that interferes with your daily activities, by causing difficulty in rising from a chair and sitting down, getting in and out of the car, or climbing up and down stairs. You might think that as long as you avoid a specific movement, you won't have any pain. Of course, little by little, you start adding to the list of activities to avoid until, finally, your life is restricted to a few, limited things you can do without pain.

Even a very active person can have similar problems. A small musculoskeletal imbalance or weakness can significantly limit an active individual's ability to perform at an optimum level. It can even result in your changing a favorite mode of exercise due to pain. No matter how hard you train or modify your technique, you can't seem to rise above the plateau. For example, at the third mile in a run your knee begins to hurt, or you can't play golf anymore because you will be laid up the next day with back pain. For the more elite athlete, an inability to cut, jump, balance, or accelerate as well with one side of the body greatly affects performance.

Peter, an up-and-coming triathlete, came to see me because he was unable to log the training miles from biking and running that he needed to improve his competition times. Sure, he could run ten miles and feel okay or bike thirty miles and feel pretty good, but as soon as he crossed those thresholds, his body began to break down, and the pain in his hip forced him to stop. Peter could swim without a problem, but that was only one third of what a triathlete needs to do. At the ten-mile run and the thirty-mile bike, Peter's body could no longer tolerate the stress that his training put on it. His mechanical deficiencies became magnified, and pain reared its ugly head. So, running or biking was not the problem; it was the way Peter ran and biked. The program we designed for him reeducated his body to move the way it was supposed to move, without the mechanical stress that it was so accustomed to. Peter is now competing at a level he never thought possible, and without pain. He is a winning example of how body mechanics must first be viewed from a macro level. Although he's a competitive athlete, Peter still had to begin with the fundamentals just like everyone else. If he hadn't started with the basics, his body would have resorted to its old familiar ways.

The Path to Pain

To help you understand what caused your present condition, I'd like to take you through what I term the "Path to Pain." Everyone's path is unique, but there is a sequence of events that's common to individuals whom I see in private practice. It isn't unique to the people who come to Function First; it happens to almost everyone. It's a series of events that, when traced back, often leads us to the underlying cause of an individual's pain. As you read, you'll begin to understand how this applies to you, and more than likely, to many people you know. You will not discover something extraordinary and unique; instead, you and your "healing team" (doctors, therapists, chiropractors, etc.) will begin to place emphasis on long-term rehabilitation and the prevention of future occurrences by looking beyond each symptom and seeking the underlying mechanical trigger.

In my opinion, the Path to Pain begins with muscle imbalance issues. A muscle imbalance is a discrepancy in length and strength between two opposing muscle groups. That is, muscles that oppose each other (pull in opposite directions) need to maintain a mutually beneficial relationship. They should have corresponding lengths and strengths that allow a joint to move equally and within its normal range of motion. A predictable pattern occurs with these muscle imbalances based on how our neurological system works. It's a dirty little trick that our bodies play on us. You see, when a muscle gets tight, it begins to demand more attention from our command center, the central nervous system (CNS). The tight muscle thus receives more of the information from the CNS, until it deprives the opposing muscle of its fair share of the information. This is equivalent to adding fuel to the fire. The shorter, tighter muscle continues to get even shorter and tighter. The opposing muscle now becomes long and weak as a result. Therefore, the situation perpetuates itself, if you do not recognize and act upon it. Ultimately, these muscle imbalances will result in altered or inappropriate movement patterns, which are precursors to many types of musculoskeletal injuries.

Muscle imbalances can be caused by many different things. The most easily recognized are those associated with habitual postures. For many people, the picture of a slouching teenager may come to mind. When left unaddressed, these postures become more ingrained in people's physical characteristics. Other examples of habitual postures are a tendency to always stand on one leg or to regularly shrug the shoulders in response to cold, fear, or tension. Women who were teenagers and young adults in the 1950s and 1960s were taught to tuck their buttocks under when they stood. Over time, this affects the position of the pelvis and the lower back. Habitual postures can also develop from psychological influences. Certain observable postures are often associated with depression and fatigue, others with stress and fear. A person who consistently experiences these emotions may reinforce these undesirable postures.

Another major cause of muscle imbalances is the work environment. If you do a lot of any one thing, your body will get stronger and more efficient at the mechanics it takes to complete that task. This can lead to tighter and stronger muscles associated with accomplishing that movement. This is true whether you use a computer or run a jackhammer every day. If you sit all day with your hands in front of you, certain muscles will likely develop tightness, while their antagonist muscles will develop weakness. The same principle applies if you always hold a particular work tool the same way or have to assume a specific stance on a regular basis (e.g., as a grocery checker).

Past injuries and surgeries can also cause muscle imbalances. Trauma to the body, be it from an accident or surgery, creates a response within the tissue. This includes the skin, the fascia, the blood vessels, the ligaments, the muscles, and the nerves. But we all knew this, right? You've experienced this if you fell and skinned your knee or your buttocks became bruised from a needle. For the sake of our discussion, however, the importance of this response to the tissue is how it affects the way we move. If there is a lack of movement in one part of the body, be it a muscle or a joint, the body will make up for it somewhere else. Let's say that you strained the hamstring muscle in the back of your left thigh. Strains come in different degrees of severity—from just a few torn muscle fibers to a complete tear, in which one side of the entire muscle is separated from the other side. So, let's say that your strain was pretty bad, and the skin above the muscle became discolored and bruised (this is due to bleeding of the damaged muscle fibers). As that tear heals, one part of the process is that the body places scar tissue in and over the region of the tear(s). Scar tissue does not have the same elastic properties that muscle has. This means that a muscle full of scar tissue does not lengthen or stretch the way a healthy one does. If left to heal on its own, that injured hamstring muscle will have less flexibility at the hip and the knee joints that it helps to move. The result is that even though the bruising has disappeared, the damage remains and can continue to impact the rest of your body.

Another way to develop muscle imbalances is through improper physical training—for example, how individuals work out in the gym, the way athletes train, and how a "weekend warrior" participates in his or her sport. The main difference between improper physical training and stressful activity in the work environment is the intensity of the former versus the duration of the latter. Work-related imbalances are often caused by repeating certain tasks and movements over a prolonged period of time. During physical training, muscle imbalances tend to develop as a result of overloading the muscles improperly—for example, a young man who spends most of his time in the gym training what I call the "mirror muscles." These are muscles that he sees in the mirror—the chest, the biceps, and the abdominals. Since he doesn't see the opposing muscles on the back side of his body, he doesn't give them the same attention. Although he may do this only two or three times a week, he is adding resistance to the body in the form of the weights he lifts. Therefore, he is making himself dysfunctionally stronger; although his toned muscles may look good, they in fact cause an overall negative impact on the body.

Another good example is a middle-aged woman who is an avid golfer. She loves to walk the course for exercise and never uses a cart. She may play only a few times a week or every two weeks, but because golf is a one-sided sport, she tends to develop detrimental muscle imbalances on one side of her body. Although she isn't working against resistance a way the weight lifter is, she has had to develop her body's muscular force to generate speed in the club to hit the ball. No matter how good a golfer she is, she would do this at least one hundred times each round, if her actual strokes plus practice swings were added up. In this example, it is the repetition of a single, one-sided movement that results in the stress.

Another type of improper physical training that can negatively impact the body is walking or running asymmetrically. Your movements should be symmetrical, from left to right. Now, many professionals in my field would probably be quick to point out that very few, if any, humans are perfectly symmetrical in their gait. Yet when the trained eye can observe asymmetries without the use of high-tech recording equipment, it's obvious that damage is being done to your body with every step. Asymmetries in your gait reveal the effects of your postural misalignments and muscle imbalances. Walking is your posture in motion. Take a look at an older pair of your running or walking shoes and see whether the wear patterns are the same on both soles. If you see exaggerated wear on the inner sole or the outer heel, you may have a problem with an asymmetrical gait. This is just one way to see firsthand the uneven wear and tear to your body. In addition, notice whether you form calluses regularly on one area of a foot that you don't form on the other foot.

The last few contributing factors to muscle imbalances are those that you have very little control over. One such type consists of congenital factors. You are born with them—for instance, having one leg slightly longer than the other. This is a "true" leg-length discrepancy. I say "true," because many people have imbalances that make one leg appear longer than the other when it really is not. True leg-length discrepancy is one in which a bone or several bones are longer in one leg than in the other. This can create compensatory changes all throughout the body, as the individual adjusts to the uneven base.

Scoliosis can also (though not always) be a congenital musculoskeletal issue. Scoliosis refers to a lateral curvature of the spine. This is seen when the spine is viewed from the back. Muscles on either side of the spine that should be of the same length are instead drastically different from one side to the other. Scoliosis is also found with a leg-length discrepancy, as a way for the body to compensate for the sideways tilting of the pelvis.

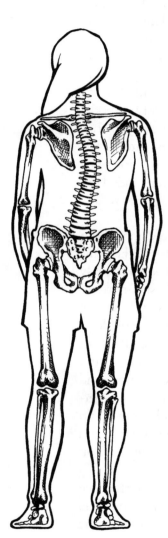

Figure 1
Woman in her early twenties with scoliosis

Other muscle imbalances develop indirectly as a result of neurological or neuromuscular disease. Examples of these would be imbalances due to stroke, Parkinson's disease, or fibromyalgia.

I'd like to make a very important point about congenital and disease-related imbalances: just because an individual wasn't directly responsible for the development of these imbalances doesn't mean that he or she is helpless to change them. To do this, we must stop the downward spiral by steering the body off the path of least resistance that it has traveled for so many years. We can accomplish this by working on getting the body as close as possible to an ideal alignment, using the exercises outlined in this book.

For example, let's look at the illustration of a woman in her early twenties who has congenital scoliosis (see figure 1). She believed that because she was born with it, she could do nothing about it and would just have to live with it. But by allowing the body to take the path of least resistance and giving in to the muscular forces acting on the scoliosis, the curves get worse and worse. In figure 2, we can see the same woman at fifty years of age. Although the curvature of her spin has deteriorated over the years, it isn't too late to begin the Function First program. The improvement in quality of life that one can experience by reversing the path of least resistance is worth every repetition of every last set of exercises.

How do you know whether you have muscle imbalances? A very effective way is to observe your static, relaxed posture. This, in itself, is not that easy for someone with an untrained eye, but in chapter 9 I'll provide you with examples of some of the more common postural faults that we regularly see. You can compare your stance with these examples in the mirror or let someone else inspect your posture and match your body to the closest example given.

The Story of Brian

Let us consider my client, Brian, who had a job loading and unloading furniture. He hurt his back because of muscular weakness throughout his core (hips, pelvis, and torso). Brian essentially stressed the muscles and the ligaments in his lower back because he wasn't strong enough to protect his spine against the outside force created by the weight of a piece of furniture. Brian's visit to the worker's compensation doctor resulted in orders to take two weeks off work, while using muscle relaxants and anti-inflammatories.

Returning for a follow-up visit two weeks later, Brian had only slightly improved symptomatically. The doctor then ordered an MRI (magnetic resonance imaging), a diagnostic tool that would determine whether any damage had occurred. It took about ten days to get an appointment and receive the MRI results. The MRI showed that Brian had a damaged disc between the vertebrae (bones) in his lower back. Depending on the extent of the damage and the philosophy and the ethics of the doctor, Brian's treatment could have gone several different ways.

A conservative-minded doctor would have sent Brian to physical therapy. Of course, at this point, he had already lived with the injury for twenty-four days, and it might even be longer before he could get physical therapy approved by his worker's compensation provider, as well as an appointment with a physical therapist. Valuable time would be lost. The longer Brian waited, the more deconditioned his body would become. The longer his pain lasted, the more likely his body would learn new coping strategies—compensations and apprehensions—to handle the pain.

Another doctor might have referred Brian to a spine specialist for further

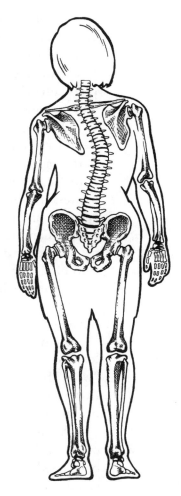

Figure 2
Fifty-year-old woman with scoliosis

evaluation. Again, more time would pass between the time of injury and proactive intervention. The spine specialist would have two options: refer Brian to physical therapy or do surgery. This is where the question of ethics and philosophy comes in. Would the spine specialist do surgery because that's what he does best? Or would he first refer Brian to a physical therapist to see whether a more conservative form of treatment might produce the desired results?

Unfortunately for Brian, he had a doctor who didn't just perform surgery; he did a spinal fusion. This involves the use of a metal "cage" to help fuse two vertebrae of the lower back together. It was not surprising to me that Brian actually felt worse after the surgery. First of all, the fusion did nothing to address the underlying cause of the injury. Second, Brian had essentially been lying around for longer than ninety days since the injury and had become terribly deconditioned.

Brian had not worked for over a year when he finally came to our Function First office. Even after the surgery, he was still in a great deal of pain and was extremely limited in the activities he could physically accomplish. Fortunately for Brian, we looked at his entire body, its condition, and what he needed to do in order to live a normal life again.

Brian started out with exercises similar to those in this book and slowly learned to use his body again the way it should be used. Instead of focusing on "what" hurt, we addressed the "why." Brian had many musculoskeletal issues that had been present before the back injury, and layers of compensation had occurred on top of the injury.

Our approach to Brian went beyond prescribing the standard "back" exercises. At this point, these exercises were actually too aggressive for Brian. His body needed an opportunity to start over. Instead of letting standard protocols guide Brian's exercise program, we let his body tell us what it could and could not do. Reproducing the pain or working "through" the pain is not part of our philosophy. The exercises that Brian received addressed muscle imbalances throughout his body and the associated movement patterns they produced. As Brian's alignment and movement patterns accepted consistent prompts from the exercises, his function improved and his pain diminished. With Function First's whole-body approach, we built a foundation for Brian to work from. Soon he was earning a living again and had renewed confidence in his body.

Brian's story illustrates the major shift that we need in current treatment models for musculoskeletal disorders. One concept that's beginning to shake things up is the idea of the "industrial athlete." This concept merges the philosophy of sports medicine with that of the workplace. The field of sports medicine has always stressed preventative screenings and active rehabilitation, with a return to activity as soon as safely possible. Preseason physicals identify risk factors for potential musculoskeletal injuries. Tightness and weakness of specific muscle groups are identified and addressed with exercise, to decrease the risk of injury.

If an athlete gets injured, therapy and intervention begin the day of the injury. The athlete doesn't make this choice; the coach does. The athlete shows up every day in the training room just as he or she would to practice. If, for example, the athlete has an ankle injury, in conjunction with ankle rehabilitation the athlete would continue with normal upper-body workouts. Instead of running, the athlete would use an upper-body aerobic device to help maintain cardiovascular fitness. Team meetings are also mandatory, so that the athlete will remain invested in the team's goals and progress.

The need for this type of philosophy in the workplace seems obvious to me. Imagine screening workers for muscle imbalances if their job responsibilities require loading and unloading trucks. Or doing a postural screening of one hundred people at an accounting firm who sit at a computer for eight to ten hours a day.

This proactive approach would have two potential benefits. The first would be an obvious opportunity to reduce the number of injuries and their associated costs. The second would signify a company's position on work-related injuries. If a worker gets hurt on the job, it's not an automatic pass for several days off work. With a physician's clearance, the worker will be back on the job, contributing to the company in any capacity that he or she can.

But how about using this model with the general public as well? The current model in both industry and the private sector typically involves a visit to the doctor. This visit might be an appointment or an unscheduled visit to the emergency room or urgent care. The doctor will diagnose the condition, provide work or life modifications (e.g., no heavy lifting, stay off that knee, etc.), and then perhaps prescribe medications. This appointment is typically followed up by a reevaluation seven to fourteen days later. Could you imagine the team doctor for a professional or an Olympic sports team telling the team's athlete to go home and come back in a week for a checkup? That doctor would be out of a job before the athlete left his office.

In the sports medicine model, the procedure would involve immediate (that day or the next) intervention by a physical therapist, an athletic trainer, or an exercise physiologist, following the guidelines provided by the treating physician. But to really break new ground in the intervention model, the evaluation and the intervention would look beyond the site of injury. This is the core concept that I profess throughout the book: intervention should affect all factors relating to the injury, both cause and effect.

Brian's is not the everyday case, but he is also not an exception. If Brian had been a professional athlete, he would not have been treated the way he was. Brian waited from 14 days to 24 days to 90 days before any outside interventions other than medications were used. Even if surgery were the only option, an athlete would be doing everything he or she could to go into and come out of that surgery as strong as possible.

The Whole-Body Approach

A study published by the National Academy of Sciences on Musculoskeletal Disorders and the Workplace concluded, "Musculoskeletal disorders should be approached in the context of the whole person rather than focusing on body regions in isolation." This means that back, neck, and shoulder pain and injuries should be traced to their underlying causes, and health-care workers should examine a patient's whole body and the way that person uses his or her body. They should not look only at the injured spot.

Brian's case is not unique in the worker's compensation arena either. This scenario is also prevalent in private insurance, especially with health maintenance organizations (HMOs). Injured people have to make their way through many "gatekeepers" before they end up in a place where help other than medication is given.

Let's consider another client whom we'll call Pat. Pat was a successful, self-employed computer graphics consultant who worked out of her home. Being self-employed, Pat did not have worker's compensation insurance, but she did have private health insurance. She spent six or more hours every day working on the computer. Pat was a forty-five-year-old female who had observable postural faults. Her personal physician diagnosed her with tendinitis of the right wrist and elbow, associated with repetitive keying on the computer. Pat's treatment plan consisted of work modifications, a prescription for anti-inflammatories, icing, and a wrist brace to wear at night to keep her wrist straight.

This is not an uncommon treatment plan. My doctor friends tell me that it's an excellent way to treat the inflammation associated with Pat's condition. I do question, however, the logic behind the plan, since this was Pat's third visit in a year with the same complaint. Yes, they were treating the inflammation, but they had not addressed the underlying reason for her recurring injury.

When Pat finally arrived at our office, it was plain to see how the mechanics of her upper body had been altered, due to the right side of her pelvis being high and her right shoulder sloping lower than the left one. Her right shoulder was unable to function the way it should have because it was so out of place; thus, she passed that responsibility on to the elbow. The elbow, doing its own work plus the work of the shoulder, was unable to provide any support for the wrist. The muscles of the wrist exceeded their work capacity. With that, the soft tissue in the area was altered, and the end result for Pat was tendinitis in the wrist. For Pat, it surfaced in the wrist, but for someone else—say, a tennis player—the pain could have been in the shoulder or the elbow.

Pat's injury would have become a continuous cycle if no one had looked beyond her wrist. Even if they had looked as far as her elbow, they would still have missed the bigger contributing factors. Pat might have ended up changing her line of work or deciding to have surgery. Surgery would have only accomplished the same objectives that her other prior treatments had: they temporarily masked the pain and did not address the cause.

Only the Proactive Need Apply

Pat and Brian were motivated people. They wanted to get better and they sought the resources to do so. As I'll say again and again, the benefits that you'll experience from your discipline and commitment will be your reward. Your efforts will result in a reduction of pain and improved function and quality of life. Your body didn't reach this point overnight, so it isn't realistic to expect an improvement overnight. Therefore, if you promise yourself to do your exercises and be committed, you can expect the benefits that accompany this program.

Now that you've taken the initiative to free yourself from pain, you must also realize that, pain or no pain, the way you've used your body for many years is a major reason why you're having problems now. To counteract your habitual movements, we have to give your body an opportunity to feel the correct way of using its muscles. The best way to do this is with exercises that teach us the basics all over again, so that we can build a solid foundation. These are not weight-lifting or aerobic exercises. They are motor-learning exercises. And as subtle as they may appear, their influence on your body will be profound.

2

A New Perspective

To grasp the origin of your pain, I feel that it's essential to have a basic understanding of the musculoskeletal system. For starters, the musculoskeletal system consists of muscles, bones, tendons, ligaments, and cartilage. And they are just that, a "system." They are all anatomically connected and functionally related. The muscles move the bones. The bones act as levers to allow the muscles to increase the amount of output or work that they are capable of. Tendons are the links between bones and muscles. They blend out of the end of a muscle and attach the muscle to the bone. Ligaments are like tendons, except that they attach bone to bone, instead of muscle to bone, to keep our skeleton connected. Ligaments don't have the same ability to stretch and recoil that a muscle has. So when they become overstretched, as with a sprained ankle, their length never returns to normal.

Associated with and intimately related to these structures is our internal computer system—the central nervous system (CNS). The CNS is the software that drives the hardware (muscles). Every good thing that the body does, like sinking the perfect putt, is dependent on the CNS coordinating all the involved muscles, producing the right amount of force, directing that force in the right direction, and then slowing down the force enough to control the follow-through. The CNS is also responsible for a lot of the bad things we do. If you're slouching as you read this, it's because the CNS isn't telling your musculoskeletal system that slouching creates long-term damage to the spine and the muscles around it. The CNS is also responsible for developing new ways to move the body when the old way or the right way no longer gets the job done. This is compensation. And with the body being so incredibly adept at compensating, we may never realize the consequences until symptoms develop.

As the previous descriptions illustrate, every part of the body truly does depend on the others. Focusing on where pain emerges will address only one small piece of the puzzle.

The knee is not, nor is any other part of the body, an entity in and of itself. The knee is merely a single variable in a very large equation. The only way to find out how the knee has been used incorrectly over the years is to look every-where *but* the knee. When I evaluate a client, my first step is to look at the joints above and below the injury. In the case of a knee, below would be the joints of the foot and the ankle, and above is the hip. Any good orthopedist or therapist would automatically include this in an evaluation. These joints have the most immediate influence over the knee, but too many good ortho-pedists and therapists stop there. This is a mistake, because many other parts of the body can have a mechanical influence on the knee, thereby altering the knee's movement.

We can identify two different types of chronic musculoskeletal pain. One type can be traced back to a specific event that initiated the pain, like a car accident or a sports-related injury. The other type can't be traced to any one event. Instead, it may have begun with minor warning signs that progressively got worse and have remained painful. Although each form of chronic pain appears to have different beginnings, they both resist resolution for similar reasons.

The person who develops chronic musculoskeletal pain that is not associ-ated with a specific event is faced with the question "Why?" Doctors and specialists probably hear this question often. If the pain originated in the mus-cles, the bones, the tendons, the ligaments, or the cartilage, the doctor would surely have identified that. And, odds are, you would have been satisfied with the answer.

Let's use the knee as an example of how we can solve the "pain" issue dif-ferently. If the cartilage is worn down on the right knee and is making bone-on-bone contact, it only makes sense that this will hurt, right? Absolutely. There is no denying that. The more critical question is, Why is the cartilage worn down on my knee?

You might receive a couple of typical responses if you get this far with your doctor. My favorite answer is when a patient is told that she has gotten older and that wear and tear have worn away the cartilage. Of course, this response doesn't explain why all of the other joints in the body feel fine and therefore must have missed a few birthdays to avoid aging at the same rate as the painful knee.

The other popular answer is that you haven't used your knee correctly over the years, which has accelerated the degenerative process. This answer begins to shed a glimmer of light on your body's mechanics. If you've gotten this far by asking "Why?" you've done better than most people. But if you continue to ask questions (e.g., "Why haven't I used my right knee correctly over the years?"), the chances of your getting a satisfactory answer significantly decrease. You may not receive a good answer because you're seeing a "specialist." This specialist may know the knee so thoroughly that he or she can perform surgery blindfolded. Perhaps the specialist's manual testing of the knee can predict what an MRI will report nine out of ten times. Yet that level of skill pertaining to one body part can cloud one's vision about the role that the rest of the body plays in the knee's mechanics. Therefore, the specialist cannot provide you with an answer if other parts of your body contributed to your knee's degeneration.

The Body's Interrelatedness

Let's take a closer look at how the rest of the body might influence the right knee that we've used as an illustration. If we observe the patient standing, instead of just lying or sitting on the examination table, we can see that the left side of the patient's pelvis is higher than the right side. And with the pelvis sloping to the right, the upper body now sits over the right leg more than over the left leg. In other words, because the left side of the pelvis is high, a greater percentage of body weight is over the right leg as compared to the left. Even with knee pain, the patient continues to put more weight on the painful side. Why? Because that's the way this woman has walked for a very long time. In fact, she has walked that way for so long, it has worn down the cartilage on the right knee, causing bone-on-bone contact. So the right knee does appear to have aged faster than the left knee, but only because the right knee has been doing its share of the work plus part of the left knee's!

The same evaluation techniques can be applied to any part of the body. Remember, we're talking about a person who has chronic pain that cannot be directly associated with any specific event or accident. The all-important point here is that this person developed chronic pain due to prolonged musculoskeletal dysfunction. The body was used inappropriately for a very long time.

Some examples of this type of dysfunction are easily recognized, once you open your eyes to other possibilities that contribute to your problems. Many of the people I help every year are amazed when they realize how interconnected the body is. Their most frequent response is, "This makes a lot of sense."

Our Self-Healing Bodies

The human organism has an amazing capacity for self-healing. Given the proper environment, our body's restoration system can heal torn ligaments, damaged nerves, broken bones, strained muscles, and so on. The best environment for recovery is that in which any stress similar to that which created the damage is removed. Would you lie out in the sun waiting for a bad sunburn to heal? No, you'd stay out of the sun so that the skin could heal and not get worse.

Interestingly, though, even in an improper, less-than-ideal environment, the body can still heal itself. But, typically, with this type of healing, proper function is compromised in the previously damaged area. For instance, imagine how a tibia (shin bone) would heal if it were never set and put in a cast. The bones would heal in the position they took as a result of the break. The leg would not only look abnormal, but it would never work the same way again. This is an extreme example of how the healing process can be less than optimal if it is not guided and nurtured. We will later see many other examples that are much less obvious, yet their consequences are equally detrimental.

The Need to Take Responsibility

I want to restate the ultimate insight that I hope you gain from this book: you have an important role in properly guiding and nurturing the healing process. We can all help this process long before we feel pain, before the doctor tells us that we require surgery, before we need medication, or before we make an appointment with a chiropractor.

If you are already in pain, don't worry. It's not too late. You see, we all are doing continuous damage to our bodies at some level, just by performing our daily activities. And the body needs to recover and heal from that damage, no matter how microscopic the damage might be.

I damaged my body today by running four miles up and down hills. Because I have good running mechanics, the damage I did to my muscle tissue was actually a good type of stress. With an appropriate recovery, which includes stretching, rehydrating, proper nutrition, and rest, I will be stronger from today's workout.

Now, if a sedentary person who hasn't run in five years does the same workout I did today and then "recovers" by coming home and flopping on the couch with a couple of cold beers, the result will be quite different. Although this individual's soreness will dissipate after three or four days, the effects of the damage will not. He may no longer be aware of the damage because the initial soreness will be gone, but another page will have been added to this person's physical history book.

As you read this book, you are a representation of all your physical experiences to date. You may have had your ups and downs, but every page that was written in your personal history book tells part of the story that led to where you are today physically. The good news is that you have an opportunity to write a happy ending.

It would be wonderful if we could just jump right to the "happy ending." But, as they often say in the social sciences, if we don't learn from our past mistakes, we're doomed to repeat them. So, we must look at the many physical issues and core beliefs that have proved detrimental to our health, well-being, and overall function.

The Role of Your Doctor

Let's begin with your doctor. Your doctor is there for you, but your doctor is not you. No doctor knows your body better than you do. When you go to the doctor with a complaint about your body, your doctor examines you, runs tests if necessary, and then applies a diagnosis to your problem. This diagnosis is based on what the doctor sees, feels with his hands, and sometimes hears. Your doctor may also come to a conclusion that's based on answers you give him to targeted questions. But your doctor can never experience what you experience. The pain, the limitations, and the inconveniences are all unique to you. There may be similarities between you and others who have like conditions, but never will their experiences be identical to yours. Therefore, this well-educated, well-meaning individual is much more limited in how he can affect your circle of influence than you realize. Nevertheless, his influence is still an important part of your route to recovery.

As figure 3 illustrates, we have immediate power over certain aspects of our health. There are some that we cannot control and yet others over which we have limited control. The graphic is based on the concepts of Stephen Covey's Circle of Influence in his book *The 7 Habits of Highly Effective People*. As you can see, the farther away you are from "You," the less influence or control you have. And the closer you get to "You," the more control you have. Things that we have the most control over should be where we spend the greatest amount of time and energy.

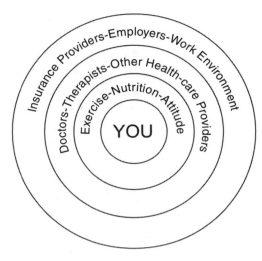

Figure 3
Illustration derived from the Circle of Influence, from The 7 Habits of Highly Effective People, *by Stephen Covey*

Once the doctor has made a diagnosis, there are four main options. He can send you to some form of therapy, prescribe medication for pain and/or inflammation, perform surgery, or do a combination of these. Once this decision has been made, the role of the doctor becomes more of an evaluator. He evaluates the impact of the intervention he prescribed and determines whether to continue, modify, stop, or apply one of the other three available options. The doctor's role becomes smaller and smaller after an accurate diagnosis has been made.

Sometimes the doctor's evaluation and your personal assessment of progress may not match, the case usually being that the doctor feels you have progressed or improved more than you think you have. This difference in opinion brings us to a critical crossroads in your history book, because if you haven't improved as much as the doctor thinks you have or should have and you're still struggling with pain, then there must be a reason. Possible reasons that might run through your mind are that the doctor made the wrong diagnosis, the prescribed drugs weren't effective, or the therapist didn't "make me well."

Perhaps it's to your advantage, as an individual seeking an improved quality of life, to consider other possibilities—possibilities outside the contemporary "menu" of options that most people adhere to. Medications top the list on this contemporary treatment menu. Just look at the profit margins of the pharmaceutical companies in this country. If medication is part of your daily regimen for coping with musculoskeletal pain, I strongly believe that it doesn't have to be.

Medications are nothing more than an adjunct to your path to a pain-free life. They are not the foundation, and they certainly aren't the ultimate answer to your problems. There isn't a single medication on earth that, by itself, relieves pain, stops inflammation, fights infections, and so on. The only way that medications can work is by helping your other bodily systems to do their jobs more effectively.

Am I telling you to flush all of your medications down the toilet right now? No. But I will give you hope and the necessary tools so that one day you should be able to do just that. This hope should inspire you to formulate a plan to get off your anti-inflammatories and pain killers. Of course, I'm going to add, "Check with your doctor first." But keep in mind that pain pills and anti-inflammatories are not life-and-death drugs, the same as, say, blood pressure medication might be. So getting off these drugs is as much your decision, if not more so, as it is your doctor's.

Falling in the same category on the menu as medication are braces and splints. Braces and splints do one of two things: (1) provide support and/or stability for a weak body part, or (2) seek to influence a positional change in a specific body part. Basically, you're asking the brace or the splint to do a job that you should be able to do yourself. And that's okay if your body needs help, especially if your ligaments lack full function and can't hold one bone to another. The brace or the splint is a means to an end, which substitutes for the deficient ligament(s). If an area is weak or unstable, you strengthen it and challenge it to increase its stability. If a body part needs to be influenced (i.e., muscle lengthening or modified movements), you make proactive changes by using your own central nervous system to create the change. By relying on your own body, you make these changes permanent and part of how your body functions.

Suppose that you go bicycling for the first time in months. You wake up the next day with incredibly sore muscles in your legs. Do you take out a pair of crutches? Of course not, because you know that your body will overcome this. It is minor damage to the tissue, due to an excess of "good stress." Essentially, the same phenomenon is happening to your bad back, your tendonitis, or your sore knee, except that these were created by an accumulation of bad stress to your body over time, which you essentially ignored until the pain began. Therefore, your recovery may have never occured because the bad stress continued to accumulate.

Taking Charge

Before you can implement any of the ideas and the exercises in this book, you have to put a whistle around your neck and take over the position of head coach. I use the term *coach* purposely because I feel that you need to look at your body and your path to freedom from pain as a team dynamic.

Your team is made up of your feet, knees, hips, back, shoulders, neck, and head. Essentially, your team consists of every part of your functioning body.

As the head coach, you need to surround yourself with a support staff of talented individuals who complement one another. These are the assistant coaches, the practitioners you choose to help prepare your team for the big game—in this case, your treatment and recovery. They are your doctors, therapists, chiropractors, acupuncturists, and so on.

Keep in mind that they are still only your assistant coaches. For example, a football team is made up of many different positions (running backs, linemen, wide receivers, etc.). Each position has a coach who knows that part of the game better than the head coach does. But the head coach is still key because he has to understand how all of the different positions work together to produce the best results for the team. Does that mean you have to go out and get a degree in anatomy? No, but you do need to manage the various members of your team and determine what's best for you.

The point is, none of your doctors or therapists know your body better than you do—so you must become an informed consumer. Putting all of your faith in one practitioner is like putting all of your savings into one stock on Wall Street. If things go well, there's nothing to worry about. But as soon as something goes wrong, your options are severely limited.

To grasp my point, look at the following table. How many squares do you see?

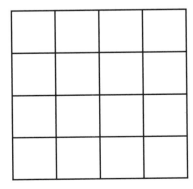

Did you say 8, 16, or 24? You may be surprised to hear that all of these are incorrect. There are actually 30 squares, including the one big square that encompasses the smaller squares.

The difference between the person who sees 16 squares and someone who sees 30 illustrates the difference between a person who never consults anyone except the family doctor and someone who plays an active role in his or her own well-being. Seeing only 16 squares and stopping there means that you were content with what was immediately obvious to you. A man wakes up in the morning, and his shoulder pinches and hurts. He attributes it to too much painting the day before. He takes some ibuprofen for the pain. Folks, this is *not* what I mean by playing an active role in your health—and going to your doctor for the same pain pills isn't any better.

Uniquely You

The body is a highly integrated unit. We are much more than the sum of our parts. In general, we all start out as infants with the same equipment. Certain individuals are given more of an opportunity to challenge themselves than others are, because their body parts are not up to "factory specifications." Others were born with fully functioning parts that later were affected by accidents or traumas. Unfortunately, most people aren't aware of the need to stimulate the different systems of the body to keep it running optimally.

As a result, there are innumerable variations between people in the functioning of their musculoskeletal systems. Even with these variations, we still must have a "gold standard," or a "blueprint," that we strive for. Of course, not everyone will be able to achieve the gold standard, but the closer we come to that standard, the more functional our bodies will be. And with improved function come improved health and well-being.

3

Picture Perfect

Have you ever noticed that the anatomical charts hanging in your doctor's office or displayed in textbooks all look alike? That's how we're supposed to look. It is the gold standard, the most mechanically effective and physiologically efficient standing position or posture. One of the best criteria for evaluating the body as a whole is to consider the standing posture. When we evaluate an individual's relaxed, natural posture, we gain insight into how that person's body functions as a whole—not how one or two specific parts function, but how the interdependent parts interact within the entire mechanism. Postural alignment is the basis of our movement patterns. If the basis of our movement begins from a less-than-optimal position, then movement itself will likely be less than optimal. Optimal standing posture, the "blueprint," has many benefits for our bodies. First of all, it enables us to neutralize the downward pull that gravity constantly exerts on our bodies. If all of the building blocks that make up our bodies were stacked on top of each other the way we were designed, gravity couldn't create pulls and torques on our tissue. To illustrate this, note the stress that is placed on your lower back when you bend at the waist to a 45-degree angle, versus what you feel when you stand up straight (figure 4). Granted,

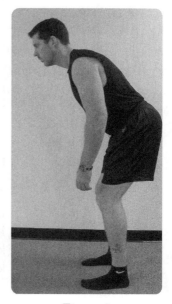

Figure 4
Bending to a 45-degree angle

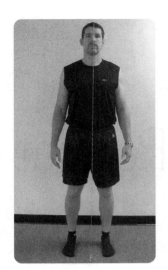

Figure 5
Plumb line front view

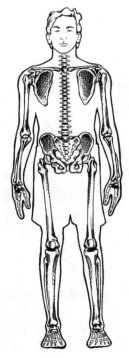

Figure 6
Blueprint front view

this is an exaggerated example and is merely used to demonstrate the effect. Now imagine being asked to walk around for ten minutes while bent at the waist to a 45-degree angle. This same effect happens on a daily basis. It's not as dramatic, but it does consistently occur. So, instead of feeling stress in your lower back for a few seconds as you bend over to 45 degrees, your body becomes accustomed to lower-grade, omnipresent, almost background stress. And just because you don't feel it every day, that doesn't mean the damaging stress has gone away. Your body is still performing acts that will contribute to long-term damage.

Look at figure 5. A plumb line is used as a reference point. The plumb line will always hang in the direction that gravity pulls. The plumb line is placed between the subject's feet to divide his base of support in half. In our blueprint (figure 6), notice how all of the body's critical weight-bearing joints are directly lined up over each other. Notice that the pelvis, the platform on which the upper body sits, is level. Notice how the spine sits directly in the center of the body and is straight when viewed from the front or the back. If the spine were to continue on down to the floor, it would land dead center between the two feet. The head sits on top of the spine and is therefore centered perfectly on the body. The shoulders are of equal height, and the arms hang the same distance from the body on either side, with the palms facing in. The only additional area to note is the shoulder blades in the back. The inside borders of the shoulder blades should run parallel to the spine.

Now look at figures 7 and 8. Our blueprint, when viewed from the side, also shows the proper positioning of those weight-bearing joints stacked on top of each other. See how the plumb line runs from the ankle up through all of the body's weight-bearing joints. The placement of the shoulders and the head are also directly in line. Take note of the soft "S" curve that's present in the spine. Having the right amount of inward and outward curves in the spine keeps the upper body positioned properly over the lower body and keeps the head sitting directly over the shoulders.

Proper postural alignment allows for our joints' contacting surfaces to line up exactly as they should. All of our joints have one side that matches the other, enabling them to move together.

Some examples would be the ball and socket that make up your hip and shoulder joints or the hinge design of your knee and elbow joints. When the proper relationship between the two sides is maintained, the joint can move freely through its designed range of motion (ROM). If the muscle or the connective tissue on one side of the joint pulls more than do those on the other side, which can be caused by muscle imbalances, the proper relationship of the two sides is not maintained. Instead, the range of motion in one direction becomes greater, and the range of motion in the other direction decreases. Should this happen, your joint(s) lose normal movement, which prompts the body to figure out another way to perform a task. Unfortunately, the "other" way is typically detrimental to the health of our muscles and joints. Proper joint alignment also reduces the joints' susceptibility to wear and tear, because each entire joint is being used the way in which it was designed. Therefore, isolated portions of each joint's surface don't absorb the brunt of the work, and stress is better distributed throughout these areas. Just as a car's tire that makes full contact with the road lasts much longer than does a misaligned tire, the joint that is properly lined up will remain functional and pain-free longer than a misaligned joint will.

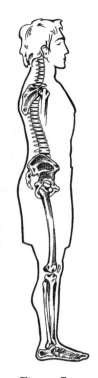

Figure 7
Blueprint side view

What Your Posture Tells You about Your Body

There is an important distinction to make between standing or static posture and what it means to be functional and pain-free. Standing posture is a "snapshot" of how the many components of your musculoskeletal system work together. Static posture is a reflection of four very important elements of the neuromusculoskeletal system (your nerves, muscles, and bones):

1. muscle balance
2. kinesthetic sense
3. neuromuscular coordination
4. mechanical efficiency

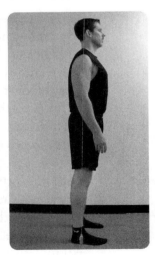

Figure 8
Plumb line side view

Each of these is interdependent and is essential to good musculoskeletal function, optimal health, and pain-free living.

1. *Muscle balance.* Every muscle in your body exists for a reason. There are no "extras" or accidental misplacements. Each muscle is responsible for specific movements, and each muscle has a counterpart called an antagonist. For every bicep, there is a tricep. In other words, if there is a muscle or muscles that bend the elbow, then there is also a muscle or muscles that straighten the elbow. In proper postural alignment, opposing muscle groups have a mutually respectful arrangement. They maintain an equal degree of pull on either side of a joint, and they share essential information from the nervous system. This allows the joint to move with equal efficiency and freedom in every direction that it is designed to move. The opposite is true if muscles on one side of the joint are dominant. Those muscles would be shorter and tighter. A short, tight muscle will demand more information from the nervous system. This, in turn, inhibits the antagonistic muscle(s) on the other side of the joint. An inhibited muscle will eventually become longer and weaker to allow for the needs of the shorter and tighter muscle. For example, if the muscles of the chest are worked all the time and they become short and tight, they'll inhibit the muscles between the shoulder blades. This pulls the joint that those muscles act upon out of alignment, causing the shoulders to round forward. As mentioned earlier, this will lead to abnormal movement patterns and excessive wear and tear on various structures in the body.

2. *Kinesthetic sense.* This term means our innate spatial awareness of our bodies, movements without the use of visual aids. Kinesthetic sense, or kinesthesia, applies to the location and the rate of the movement. For example, if I stand with my eyes closed and raise my right arm straight out to the side, then bend my elbow to 90 degrees, I still know exactly where my hand is in space. I know this from the change in length and the tension of certain muscles in my arm. Therefore, a person with good kinesthetic sense should be aware when the posture of his or her body is improperly aligned. The converse to this is a person who has bad postural alignment and is unaware of it. This person has poor kinesthetic sense. Nothing more clearly illustrates this than when our clients first see pictures of themselves standing behind a plumb line with a background grid. Although they may look at themselves every day in the mirror, they never view their bodies from this perspective. Once they see the deviations from the "blueprint," they are stunned. Many cannot believe that they hold their bodies so out of alignment on a daily basis. The pictures clearly show that a shoulder is much

lower, the body has shifted to one side, or the head is tilted. Yet these people, who have looked at themselves in the mirror every day of their lives, have never seen their misalignment until shown the images from this perspective.

One way to test your kinesthetic awareness is to close your eyes and try to touch the tips of your index fingers together in front of your face. If you touch tip to tip, you have pretty good kinesthetic sense. If you'd like to make the test a little harder, try the same thing by touching your fingertips behind your head and see how you do.

3. *Neuromuscular coordination.* In clinical terms, neuromuscular coordination applies to the relationship between the input and the output. The input is the information that your body gathers about the position of your parts in space relative to one another, the location of your center of gravity, and your environment. Your body has several different types of information gatherers. They are in your muscles, your joints, the skin, your inner ear, and your eyes. With faulty alignment, these information gatherers become "biased" toward inappropriate positioning of your body segments related to postural misalignment. In other words, over time your body sets a new baseline for what is "normal." Right or wrong, this becomes your standard. The output in most cases will be either movement or the need to stabilize yourself, as you would do on a rocking boat. It will be the result of how you process the input. That means coordinating certain muscles to work as the prime movers, other muscles to assist, others to neutralize, and others to turn off and do nothing. All of this is possible only if the input is accurate and the muscles and the joints are capable of doing what is requested of them. Friends of mine who are computer experts have a saying, "Garbage in equals garbage out," meaning that you can ask your processor (your central nervous system) to work only with what you give it. Have you ever seen someone walking along and not notice a step down? An individual who doesn't see changes in the environment is unable to anticipate changes in his or her support base. The person's only chance to react is after the body senses an increase in distance from the foot to the ground. Someone with good neuromuscular coordination will recover from this sudden disturbance very easily, perhaps with a little stumble. This person's neuromuscular system will have signaled the muscles throughout the body to respond to the sudden change and restore an upright position. The opposite is true for someone with poor neuromuscular coordination, who won't be able to respond quickly and effectively enough to prevent a fall or a possible injury. An interesting point about neuromuscular coordination is that it improves when

it's challenged. If you spend your day in a chair and your evenings sitting in front of the television, your body becomes less efficient at responding to your needs. This has serious consequences for someone who doesn't take action to recover from an injury, because the predisposition toward reinjury grows even greater.

4. *Mechanical efficiency.* As mentioned earlier, postural alignment is the basis for movement patterns. You cannot have optimal movement if your alignment is faulty. The same mechanical laws that apply to any piece of machinery also apply to the human body. Imagine a Mercedes-Benz, the pride of German engineering. Now, imagine that we take that Mercedes apart, piece by piece. Then we put it back together but don't remember where all of the parts go. They all end up somewhere, but not exactly where they're supposed to be. Do you think this Mercedes-Benz will still be an engineering marvel? Not likely. And such is the case with movements that we perform when they originate from a dysfunctional foundation. This applies as much to the way you use a keyboard as it does to how you run up a flight of stairs.

These four elements of the neuromusculoskeletal system must function properly in order for you to avoid damaging stress to your body. And if they don't, your posture will reveal what has gone wrong.

If static posture provides us with an overall "snapshot" of the body's level of function, then a person's gait gives us a moving picture. Human gait, or one's way of walking, is really posture in motion. By observing the way a person walks, we can often confirm many of the things we see in static posture. Yet, a person's gait can sometimes reveal additional problems that were hidden when he or she stood still.

Have you ever noticed that from a distance, you can often identify someone you know by the way that person walks? The characteristics that we note about certain people are a reflection of the mechanical strategies that they use to walk. Just as with static posture, we can define "normal" gait. As the body deviates from its normal gait, the likelihood of increased stress and strain on the soft tissue and the bony structures is greater. There are too many combinations of possible deviations to count, but I'm sure you're aware of the more obvious and common ones. For instance, some people are rounded forward in their upper backs with their heads forward. Others display the "duck walk," in which one or both feet turn out. There is also a type of walk associated with runway models, in which the hips swivel from side to side. Even these few, simple examples are evidence of an improper gait pattern.

You might say to yourself, "I've walked this way or stood this way all of my life, long before I started having problems." Or, "Of course, I stand or walk this way; this is what pain has done to me." In both cases, your observations are right, and in both cases, your body is wrong. What this means is that whether your structural misalignment and gait problems are a cause or an effect, it matters much less than you might think. The reality is that your body is doing something wrong on a day-to-day basis that is detrimental to your health and quality of life. So, whether it's a cause or an effect is secondary to the fact that it's now an existing part of how you move and function.

How Some Problems Might Start

Let's look in more detail at some major contributing causes to deviations in our structure. Most people are affected by more than one cause, and several of the causes can often develop as a result of the others. The major causes of structural deviations are (1) past injuries and/or surgeries, (2) congenital conditions, (3) improper physical conditioning, (4) work environments, (5) habitual postures, and (6) muscular dysfunctions/disease.

We'll use the issue of past injuries or surgeries to illustrate a point. There probably isn't a person on earth who hasn't had some minor bodily injury at one time or another during his or her life. Especially as children and during our developmental teen years, we experience countless minor strains, sprains, bumps, and bruises. We also get weekend warrior–type injuries, in which a guy or a gal who doesn't move all week tries to play as hard as possible on the weekend. The weekend warrior often participates only on the weekend because the individual needs the rest of the week to recover. Most of these injuries may hurt enough for the person to self-medicate, but they aren't severe enough to prompt a trip to the doctor.

In addition to these minor pains, many people experience more significant injuries, due to accidents or traumas, that require appropriate treatment by qualified health-care professionals. The ultimate intervention by a health professional would be surgery. Remember, all of your physical experiences to date define who you are from a musculoskeletal standpoint. Therefore, all of these incidents were and are capable of influencing how your body works now.

The first issue with either an injury or a surgery is the actual damage that's done to the tissue in the immediate vicinity of the injury. Whenever there is an insult to soft tissue (a sprain, a strain, inflammation, an incision, a contusion, etc.), a disruption occurs in the normal characteristics of that tissue. It needs to be repaired. The body can usually do this on its own, over time, unless there is a complete tear. If that's the case, surgery is typically required to reattach the two ends. The severity of the damage, of course, determines how much change will occur. There is a distinct difference in the damage associated with a surgery that neatly cuts through several layers of muscle and that which occurs with a minor muscle strain. If we're talking about damaged muscle, the particular area of damage doesn't completely return to pre-injury status. As part of the healing process, the body lays down connective tissue in the area that is supposed to have muscle tissue. However, connective tissue doesn't have the same stretch and recoil properties as muscle tissue. The result is a muscle that isn't 100 percent repaired. How close one can get to 100 percent is directly related to the steps that are taken after the injury. If we're talking about ligaments, they never had the stretch and the recoil properties of a muscle in the first place. They're like a piece of stretched gum—it doesn't snap back but stays stretched. This isn't a good situation, considering that the primary responsibility of a ligament is to connect a bone from one side of a joint to a bone on the other side of the joint. The ligament helps guide the movement of the joint, which is created by the muscle contraction. So, if your ligaments are stretched, you have a loose, floppy joint. Then you have to rely solely on your backup stabilizers for that joint: the muscles.

What I've just described can very easily be associated with specific events in one's life—events such as falls in the playground, injuries during a sporting event, car accidents, and so on. But many of these traumas also happen every day, and we just don't realize it. They are background-type, low-level insults to the tissue, which can be referred to as chronic, low-grade sprains or strains. This type of injury can happen as you hunch over your computer for eight hours a day. It can happen due to the way you walk or even how you stand in line at the grocery store. It's a cumulative effect that prompts the body to respond the same way that it does to a more definitive event, like spraining your ankle. The body's response is to begin laying down connective tissue to help protect the injured area, which results in stiffness in the muscles and the joints; this, in turn, leads to a restricted range of motion in the joints. These effects just happen more slowly and over a longer period of time.

What's really dangerous about this type of low-grade sprain or strain is that it sneaks up on you. No specific event has brought it on, so you don't remember when it arrived. And once it arrives, you don't really know it's there. As the condition progressively starts to break down your body, you simultaneously begin to build a tolerance to it. It's like living near the freeway and eventually never hearing the cars anymore. This background problem can often be directly associated with other ailments that you might seek help for, but because you don't know the problem exists and the symptom is somewhere else, you cannot make a connection between the background noise and the symptom. Many of my clients are heavy computer users because of the role that computers play in our society. I can often look at them and see where the shoulder muscles will be very tight and tender. When I ask my client whether their shoulders are sore, they say, "No." Yet, if I use my thumb to put a little pressure in that area, they jump out of their chairs. My thumb is kind of like an occasional police siren that reminds them that they do live near the freeway.

This background insult to the tissue is created by the force of gravity acting on a misaligned body. Remember, when proper postural alignment is maintained, the body is very effective at neutralizing the downward pull of gravity. The opposite is true if we aren't properly aligned, and this will be reflected in activities that we perform both statically (like sitting) and dynamically (like walking or dancing).

Like a Pebble Dropped in a Lake

Now let's take an in-depth look at the ripple effect of an injury to your body. Consider that when you have an injury, new or old, the body does what it can do to avoid pain. Minor adjustments, when looked at individually and for an isolated period of time, don't seem like a big deal. Yet something as common as a sprained ankle, if not rehabilitated properly, can lead to changes throughout your body. Intuitively, the body limps to avoid placing too much weight on the injured body part. As you do this for a few weeks, your body begins to learn this new way of walking. As a result, changes occur in the muscles that act on the knee, the hip, and the trunk. Another example may be a problem with the rotator cuff of the shoulder. If certain movements produce pain, such as reaching overhead, you'll avoid them. But if you need to get that arm overhead, you may compensate by "hiking" the shoulder toward the ear. After repeating this movement for several weeks, you wouldn't even be aware that you're shrugging the shoulder. That's because you've taught your shoulder a new incorrect way of operating, through repetition.

Vladimir Janda, M.D., an expert in the area of muscle balance, calls this phenomenon sensory motor amnesia. Your body forgets how to move properly. In our context, properly means functionally. Your body has replaced the old movement pattern of raising your arm by the ball-and-socket joint with the added movement of hiking up your shoulder blade. Even after your surface injury heals in the rotator cuff, your body will keep part of the movement that it learned while in pain. Is there a problem with this? Absolutely, because this newly learned movement actually predisposes the same shoulder to a reinjury. In addition, it can create an entire series of new problems that relate to the new dysfunction. For example, the muscles that hike up the shoulder will continue to get stronger and will compensate for other muscles. Potential problems could arise in the neck, the elbow, and the wrist on the same side of the body. This illustrates precisely how the pages of the history book that make up your physical experiences are written.

I'm sure that most of this sounds foreign to you. You have always moved along just fine, going about your workday or exercise program. This is the body that has gotten you through all the years of growing up, earning a living, and so on, and now I'm telling you that you're doing it all wrong! How could you have gotten this far if you were, in fact, doing everything wrong?

We can never test drive another human body. We cannot step outside of our own musculoskeletal systems and into another to experience how it feels to do something differently. We assume that we're doing it correctly because we have only one point of reference—our own bodies. Unless you are a high-level, competitive athlete, you probably haven't paid much attention to the mechanics of the way you move. You don't think about these things until something hurts.

Quite simply, our bodies are smarter than we are. Our bodies will get from Point A to Point B the best way they know how. And if for some reason that best way doesn't work because of a tight muscle, an injury, a bruise, inflammation, or a thousand other scenarios, the body will figure out another way to get there. Compensation is the name of the game, and the human body is a world champion at it.

There are broad ends of the spectrum with respect to how much change is needed to do the things that we do. At one end of the spectrum may be an individual who was affected by polio as a child. Poor muscular development has disrupted the ability to walk properly. Now grown up, the person has figured out a way to move from one place to another. At the other end of the spectrum is someone walking barefoot on sharp gravel. The individual will have to alter his or her walk to avoid distributing body weight over small areas on the bottoms of the feet. You have probably done this yourself. Similar situations happen when the weather gets warmer and people go barefoot for the first time that season. The bottoms of the feet are soft from a winter of wearing shoes. When we walk on the hard, rough asphalt for the first time, we don't stop and think, "I'd better walk flat-footed so that I don't scrape the bottoms of my feet." Instead, our brains get new information from the bottoms of our feet telling us that we're no longer walking on Berber carpeting. We automatically, without thinking, bend slightly at the knees and the hips so that our feet flatten to better distribute the pressure from the ground over the soles of the feet.

Altering your movements once or twice, as described earlier, won't influence your body to move differently. But if it's done repeatedly over a long period of time, as in the aftermath of an injury, your body will be changed. The end result of all these little adaptations and changes is that your body will develop a new strategy to accomplish certain tasks. Whether or not the new strategy is functionally correct is another story. As we repeatedly carry out an action, it becomes "normal" for us. Unfortunately, normal in this case is not in the best interest of our long-term health. We establish a baseline from which we work, and like a carpenter whose first baseline measurement is off, it's inevitable that the rest of the project will be detrimentally affected.

4

Breakdown of the Mechanical Miracle—You!

If we are the product of all our physical experiences to date, I'd like you to take a moment to think back over the years to the major and the minor injuries your body has sustained. Try to remember as many as you can, because they all play a role in who you are today. Do you recall that sprained ankle during high school cheerleading or that deep-thigh bruise from a pickup football game back in college? They all had some effect on your body. Remember, we are all affected by both large and small injuries, so don't forget the ingrown toenail that hampered you for two weeks back in 1988.

If you are and were very physically active in sports or because of your occupation, you have a greater probability of experiencing more insults to your working machinery than does someone who leads a more sedentary life. Major injuries that require a prolonged recovery process will obviously have a greater impact on your body than a bump or bruise would. For instance, reconstruction of the anterior cruciate ligament (ACL) in your knee can take twelve or more weeks to rehabilitate. During that twelve-week period of using crutches and limping, your body learns a new motor program for movement. That is, the body has to learn to walk during this time, taking into consideration that one link in the chain from foot to hip is both unstable and lacking a full range of motion. In addition, it's also very painful to put weight on the leg, and the body doesn't like pain—so you avoid it. This also contributes to alterations in the way you walk, in an effort to avoid the pain.

On the positive side, if the rehabilitation and the follow-up for an injury like this are ideal, then the long-term implications are lessened. That's a big "if," however, because standard physical therapy protocols for a repaired ACL tend to focus predominantly on the knee. In some cases, the ankle below and the hip above the injured knee may be included in the rehabilitation process. Rarely is anything ever done to address the changes that the muscles of the torso must make to compensate for the problems of one of its locomotor apparatuses (a fancy way of saying "leg"). Nor does it address the increased demand that the other leg had to assume as a result of a prolonged period of asymmetrical (one-sided) weight bearing.

An interesting observation to note is the difference between the rehabilitation and the recovery of a professional athlete versus that of an ordinary person. One of the most noticeable differences is the recovery time. Often professional and even college athletes can return to full competition in one-half or one-third the amount of time that you or I might take just to stop walking with a limp. How do they do this? Well, for starters, they are in excellent physical condition prior to the injury. Their bodies are therefore better prepared to handle the demands of aggressive rehabilitation. *Aggressive rehabilitation* is the key phrase here. *Aggressive* refers to both the amount and the intensity of rehabilitation. An athlete who injures his or her back, for example, should return to action with a back that is stronger and more flexible than it was before the injury. Professional athletes, as well as their employers, have a monetary interest in their recovery and ability to get "back on the job." Money is definitely a motivator, but so is the fact that these individuals are achievers, and they feed off their successes.

Thus the injured athlete has a new, temporary, full-time job: fixing his or her body. It isn't unusual for professional athletes who are recovering from injuries to spend three, four, or five hours in the training room and the weight room *every* day! They are doing everything possible to maximize their bodies' healing potential—and *they* are doing the work. Certain things may be done to them by trainers and medical staff, who also provide guidance, but they must work on themselves extensively. Compare this kind of rehabilitation schedule (and its recovery time) to that of the injured individuals who might spend three hours a week rehabilitating themselves. The monetary incentives may not be the same, but the desired outcome is. Both professional athletes and injured workers want pain-free bodies that allow them to do both their jobs and all of the other things in life they enjoy. Therefore, an important question to ask yourself is, "How much time do I spend working on myself?" Please keep in mind that I refer to physically addressing the biological you, not to arguing with insurance company representatives, scheduling office visits, sitting in the waiting room, or any of those necessities. Unfortunately, these tasks are often huge time vacuums, but they still don't count toward the concrete time you must spend working on yourself. The time that you work on yourself is far more important than anything a "customer service" representative could ever do for you.

Having read up to this point, you may have started to revise your overall perspective on your physical situation. If so, that's great. Breaking through inertia is the first step. If you still aren't buying into the views I've presented thus far, please continue reading. For thirteen years, I've used this approach to help people who had no hope, so I know that this program can help you achieve freedom from pain.

Tina's Story

If you're a chronic pain sufferer, whether or not your pain is related to trauma, consider the possibility that biomechanical issues existing prior to any accident may be impeding the healing process. I think it's safe to say that your body didn't get into its present condition overnight.

Such was the case with Tina, a twenty-nine-year-old professional chef. Tina was the unfortunate driver of a car that was blindsided in an intersection by another car running a red light. The accident left her with pain on the side of her neck and down into her shoulder blade, like a "knitting needle" being stuck in her back. Prior to seeing me, Tina spent a year and a half receiving care from several chiropractors, as well as physical therapy and massage treatments. According to her, she was about 30 percent improved, but she still had a lot of pain and had a hard time working. After evaluating Tina, I pointed out to her several misalignments of her shoulders and pelvis and explained how they contributed to her pain. Interestingly, Tina responded by saying that she had been like that long before the car accident. She even brought in pictures from eight years earlier, when she was in college. She was right, she had been misaligned in terms of her posture, but the goal of her exercise program was to correct that anyway, because the postural imbalances wouldn't allow her to heal properly. Within four weeks, Tina was another 30 percent better, and in nine weeks, she was at 90 percent improvement. Today Tina is pain-free, and if she continues with her exercise program, she'll remain so long into the future.

The Unholy Trinity

I'd like to outline a series of events that happens to many individuals who currently suffer from chronic musculoskeletal pain. They are what I consider the three preliminary steps to developing long-term musculoskeletal issues—an unholy trinity, if you will. As you read, think back and see whether they apply to the process you've experienced.

The first is denial. Whether you crashed on your motorcycle or developed shoulder pain while working on the computer, you deny to yourself the seriousness and the relevance of the injury. Of course, you're aware that you're injured, especially if you crashed on a motorcycle. You may even be intellectually aware that you'll be faced with a recovery period, but unless you've ever had a prior injury that required similar attention, you may be oblivious to what you're in store for. When I use the term *denial*, I mean that you deny the seriousness of the injury and the level of effort that will be necessary on your part to effectively recover. So often, people equate this new injury with much less serious ones they've experienced in the past, saying that it's "no big deal," or that it will clear itself up in a few days or a week. Pop a few ibuprofen and take it easy for a couple of days, and things will resolve themselves, right? Wrong. Even with something more serious like a motorcycle accident, just because the swelling has decreased or the stitches have been removed doesn't mean that the healing process is complete. Many times, when individuals now must deal with chronic conditions resulting from earlier injuries, they'll look back to the initial injuries and realize that they hadn't accepted the gravity of the situation—a classic case of "If I knew then what I know now . . ."

Denial can cost you the opportunity to begin some of the most important interventions in your recovery process. If you have a clear idea of what's going on in your body, with the help of your physician or another qualified healthcare professional, you can map out a plan and know your responsibilities. This is important because, after an injury, you're working within a window of time where the body changes as a result of the injury. This is when you can influence the healing process, in order to recover to the best of your ability.

The second part of the unholy trinity is pain avoidance. Yes, I have already mentioned this earlier in one context. I said that the body doesn't like pain and does whatever possible to avoid it, but if standing for ten minutes in church causes back pain, the answer is not to avoid standing (or church). Avoiding something if it hurts might apply to thumping yourself on the head with a hammer, but it doesn't cover natural movements that the body should be able to perform. By avoiding the pain without identifying its cause, you set yourself up for additional problems down the road.

I often see people with lower-back problems who avoid activities like gardening or sitting for more than fifteen minutes because it aggravates their back pain. Or computer users who develop upper-extremity injuries associated with overuse. They will either dramatically reduce their time on the computer or manipulate their workstations temporarily to change the stress on their bodies. The reality is that they are just avoiding the pain instead of confronting it and taking the necessary steps to create an optimal recovery environment for their bodies. Eventually, any movements or activities that are similar to those that initially caused the discomfort will produce the same painful result. It's usually at this point that people decide to do something about their pain, but valuable intervention time had been lost.

The third part of the trinity is shortsightedness. I often see this situation with people who have already attempted some type of intervention or rehabilitation prior to consulting me. It usually occurs when people have stopped either physical therapy or chiropractic care because their insurance no longer covers it or else they have been discharged. Limitations on any kind of care by your insurance plan should *never* dictate the end of your rehabilitation process. Your insurance plan has no correlation with how your body heals. What happens quite often is that people discontinue any rehabilitation once their insurance no longer pays for it. It's quite possible that these individuals are still a long way from 100 percent recovery. Instead, they may be only 50 to 60 percent recovered, so they resume their normal lives within the restricted level of functioning that the 50 to 60 percent recovery allows. This is unfortunate, because an injury that could have been adequately rehabilitated within weeks, if everything were done as it should have been, may now take months or even years. It's crucial that you see the rehabilitation through to the end and do all of your homework. Don't rely on someone else to do the work for you. Others don't have the same investment in your health that you have. They don't have to climb into your skin and do what you do or feel what you feel.

When Are You Done?

When is the end of your rehabilitation? That's a great question. Perhaps a better question to ask, though, is when does your formal rehabilitation end? Your formal rehabilitation would be that dictated by a qualified professional, based on outcome objectives. You will have general time lines to follow, based on your injury and your body's capacity to heal. Now, your informal rehabilitation is another story. To me, that never ends. It's an ongoing process to fight back against the things that beat us down day after day.

I mentioned that you might get discharged from rehabilitation based on your insurance coverage. That is, your insurance might pay for only nine visits, even if your doctor wants you to go for eighteen visits. Another possible discharge scenario is when the practitioner who is treating you makes the decision. This means that either the practitioner feels he or she can do no more for you with direct intervention or, in the practitioner's opinion, you have plateaued in your improvement. Keep in mind that when a practitioner states that you've "plateaued," this simply applies to the treatment that this individual has provided for you. It doesn't mean that you cannot improve with other forms of treatment or with a consistent home program. It's perfectly acceptable and not uncommon for practitioners (at least, ethical ones) to discontinue your treatment because they feel that their skills and approach no longer benefit you. A perfect example is with chiropractic care. A chiropractor who only adjusts his or her patients and doesn't utilize any complementary stretching and strengthening programs will ultimately need the patient to do some other type of proactive work. The same can be true for a physical therapist who specializes in soft-tissue work or myofascial release, which, without complementary exercise, would have a diminishing likelihood of helping you to progress. Once again, the ball is in your court to determine what your body ultimately needs to get better.

Self-Tests

By examining the concrete examples I have used, you might see where you're having problems. However, you can also take a few simple tests to feel some of the more common movement faults that are often associated with muscle imbalances. These pertain to muscles that are tight, muscles that are weak, and muscle groups that cannot work together to coordinate proper movements.

The first is the **stork stance**, which highlights muscle weakness and balance. For this test, it's best to stand in front of a full-length mirror. Lift one foot off the ground so that your thigh is almost, but not quite, parallel to the floor. Your knee should be bent, with your foot almost behind you (figure 9). As you do this, you will watch yourself in the mirror to see what your body does. It

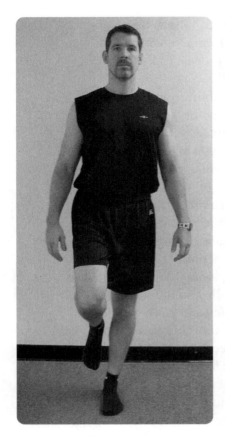

Figure 9
Stork stance

might be a good idea to try this before you read on. If you know what your body is *supposed* to do, then you might consciously or unconsciously make corrections. For some people, just standing on one foot will be a challenging task. If you are unable to balance for more than three to five seconds, then practice balancing first. Don't look at yourself in the mirror until you can balance on one foot for at least five seconds.

One way that your body might respond to this position is by allowing your torso to bend sideways toward the stance leg (the leg on which you support yourself). Or, your pelvis on the side of your stance leg might tilt up, while the opposite side drops. As this happens, your torso might bend to the side as well. You should also look at your pelvis to see if one side rotates toward the mirror as the other side rotates away. The final thing you can watch is your knee on the stance leg. Check to see whether your kneecap turns inward as you support yourself on that leg. After you have done this on one leg, repeat it on your other leg. It's very possible that you'll get different results on the other leg. Also note whether one leg feels more stable than the other.

If one or more of these movements occur, it's a reflection of weakness and lengthening of some of the important stabilizing muscles around your outer hip and pelvis. These muscles keep the pelvis in line, from side to side, when we walk, run, or go up and down stairs. We use these muscles any time we place extra weight or all of our weight on one foot at a time, as we do when walking. In addition, there should be no noticeable difference between the right and the left legs. Remember, we are a bilateral piece of machinery.

So, what should happen if your body does what it is supposed to do? First, your pelvis should remain level and your torso should stay straight up and down. In other words, you should be able to just shift your weight from two bases of support (your feet) to one base of support without any major movements in your pelvis, hips, and upper body. Therefore, your pelvis should not turn toward the mirror, nor should your knee face anywhere except straight ahead.

Our next self-test involves the **wall stance**. Stand with your back to the wall and your heels 2 or 3 inches from the wall (3 inches away at most). Allow your arms to hang at your sides. Now stand so that your head, shoulders, and buttocks all touch the wall. You will have to bring your shoulder blades toward each other to be able to get your shoulders back (figure 10).

In general, this will feel very strange and awkward for many of you. Essentially, to achieve this position, you must engage all of the extensor muscles that run up and down your spine from your pelvis to the base of your skull. Whether you can attain this position and how you do so is the insight you gain from this test.

One of the first things you might notice is that your weight is forward, on the balls of the feet. As a result, you might feel your calf muscles working harder than normal to press you back toward the wall. For some people, getting their heads on the wall is the most challenging task. When the upper back is rounded as part of one's posture, the head must go forward to balance the weight that's shifted behind the ankles. Assume this position long enough, and you won't have strength in the upper-back muscles to extend (straighten) it enough to allow the head to come all the way back. Some people may be able to get their heads on the wall but only by tipping them back. In other words, they would

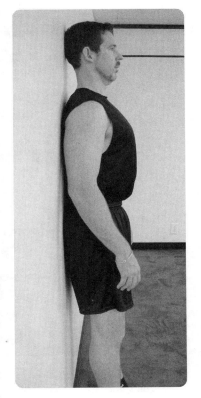

Figure 10
Wall stance

have to look up at the ceiling to get their heads to touch the wall. When the head touches the wall in this manner or doesn't touch it at all, this reveals a definite weakness in the very important muscles of the upper back.

For people who can get their heads and upper backs on the wall, there still may be concerns. Another technique used—and, yes, it's a compensation—is to exaggerate the arch in the lower back to get the shoulders and the upper back on the wall. This technique is often resorted to by people who already have a great deal of arch in their lower backs and whose abdominal strength is weak relative to their hip flexor strength and tightness. For these individuals to achieve this position, their buttocks will touch the wall but no other part of their backs will touch until their shoulder blades do. The concave arch in the back therefore extends all the way up to the shoulder blade region of the upper back (figure 11).

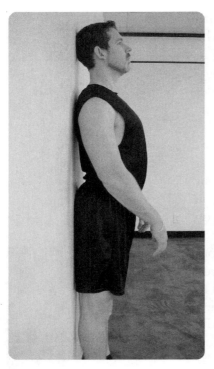

Figure 11
Wall stance with arched back

If you aren't sure whether you compensated by arching your lower back, we have a little addition to this test. It will help to reveal whether you have the necessary strength in your abdominals to keep your lower back neutral under this kind of demand.

The next step is to fold your arms in front of you. This may make your shoulders come forward a little, but you still need to keep the shoulder blades on the wall. From this position, try to press your lower back flat against the wall. As you do this, you cannot allow your head or shoulders to come off the wall or allow your knees to bend. Many people will find this very challenging. If you cannot do this, you have weakness in the abdominal and the gluteal muscles.

Next we can try the **cat and dog**. The cat and dog, sometimes called the cat and camel, is a yoga exercise, but I use it as an evaluation tool to see how well a person can integrate movements of the hip, the pelvis, the spine, the shoulder girdle, and the head. The shoulder girdle refers to the shoulder blade, the upper arm bone, and the collar bone. This is the most complex of our self-tests because it integrates so many different areas of the body.

You begin this movement on your hands and knees. Your hips should be directly over your knees, and your shoulders should be directly over your wrists. Your hands are shoulder-width apart, and the fingers should point straight ahead. Your knees are hip-width apart. It's essential that you keep your elbows straight during this entire movement. I'll explain the movement in stages, beginning at the head. However, the exercise should be done as one continuous movement and not be broken up into stages.

First, look up toward the ceiling with your head and exhale. As you do this, allow the shoulder blades to collapse together and the upper back to flatten. The stomach area, or midsection, should be completely relaxed, sagging toward the floor. This will allow the lower back to sway. The buttocks should then be sticking up in the air. The final movement for the "dog" should look like figure 12. From here, you will reverse directions. Tuck your chin toward your chest and inhale. Raise your upper back up like a "mad cat." As you do this, the shoulder blades should separate. Use your abdominal muscles to tuck your pelvis under, and this will round out the lower back as well. The final movement for the "cat"

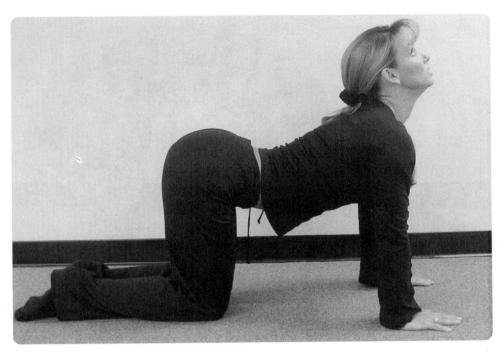

Figure 12
Dog

should look like figure 13. Following this, reverse directions again back to the "dog," where your head is up and your back is swayed.

Many things could potentially be done incorrectly with this movement. Again, let's start with the head. Are you able to coordinate the movement of your head with the rest of your body, or do you find your head going in the opposite direction from the rest of you? Are you looking down when your back is swayed or are your eyes looking up as you round your back? How about your elbows? Remember, the elbows should be straight during the exercise, in both the cat and the dog position. It is extremely challenging for people to keep their elbows straight when they allow the shoulder blades to come together as the upper back flattens. And it's very important that you are able to relax completely between the shoulder blades and allow them to drop all the way together. This won't happen if you don't effectively allow the upper back to settle completely into extension. Next, when you move between the two directions, you should be able to keep your hips over your knees from the side view. In other words, when your head is up and your back is swayed, you

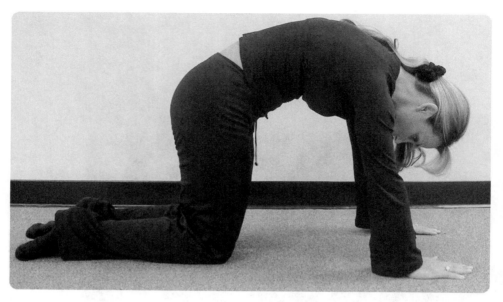

Figure 13
Cat

shouldn't shift back toward your heels. And when your head is down and your back is rounded, you shouldn't shift forward toward your hands. Another point to consider is that when you go into the mad cat, or the flexion of your spine, the spine should essentially be an evenly shaped arc. There should not be an excessively noticeable "hump" in the upper back as you do this. And there must be adequate control of the abdominal muscles to pull the pelvis under, causing the lower back to round and to keep that even arc.

Obviously, it would be most helpful to perform this exercise for your viewing purposes in front of a full-length mirror. Among the insights we get from the dynamic portion of this exercise is whether an individual has or lacks the ability to coordinate movements of the head and the pelvis. This is critical to our species as bipeds (two-legged creatures).

So, how did you do? Did you pass all the tests with flying colors? If you did, that's great, but don't get too excited. Those were just a few quick tests to help you evaluate the "basic" functioning of your musculoskeletal framework. If you didn't pass with flying colors, you are beginning to self-evaluate some of your personal musculoskeletal deficits. This is an essential step in taking control of your own recovery and finding success with this program. As the book progresses, I'll present more opportunities for you to self-evaluate and heal.

5

The Physical Laws of Our Bodies

Regardless of the pain or the type of job or incident that is associated with the pain, certain irrefutable physical laws affect our bodies. For instance, there are laws that apply to how muscles are arranged and how joints are designed to work. Certain laws also guide how our bodies gather information from the environment, how we use that information, and how our bodies respond to good and bad stress. Breaking the law has repercussions— the aches and the pains that this book addresses. The only way to avoid breaking the law is to first know the law.

Death and taxes are not the only things guaranteed in life. Gravity is right there with them. Gravity, the force that we associate with the apple falling from the tree and hitting Sir Isaac Newton on the head, is both our friend and our foe.

How important is gravity? As an individual in pain, consider this: If you lived in the water or on the moon, you probably wouldn't have many musculoskeletal problems. In both of these places, the force of gravity is reduced to an insignificant degree. That equates to less stress on the bones, the joints, the tendons, and the ligaments. The other side of the coin is that without gravity, our bones would weaken and our bodies' key information gatherers regarding movement, called proprioceptors (we'll discuss these in more detail later), become much less effective.

Most of us won't travel to space any time soon; however, similar effects can be seen with prolonged disuse of the musculoskeletal system. An obvious example would be someone who requires bed rest for one or more weeks. This person would not be able to adequately challenge his or her musculoskeletal system even with the movements of daily living. Yet a much less obvious example is probably applicable to many of you: the lack of stimulation that our "antigravity" muscles receive when we go from the bed to the car, to the desk, to the car, to the stationary bicycle, to the car, to the recliner, and then finally back to bed. These "antigravity" muscles, such as the spinal erectors or the gluteals, are a key part of the body's infrastructure. It is mandatory for an upright species that these muscles do their job. Unless we're lying down or sitting supported, we have to resist the gravitational pull of earth on our bodies to remain erect. This requires work by our muscles, which is precisely the reason we cannot sleep standing up the way that some four-legged animals can. As with any other unused or unchallenged muscles, the antigravity muscles weaken and atrophy. If they do weaken, we are haunted by that "C" word again—*compensation*. Other muscles may try to do the best they can to help out, but the outcome will never be the same. Once again, the compensation will lead to changes in the way our joints line up and how and when our muscles pull, as well as which muscles pull. Each of these factors predisposes us to injury and creates a potential barrier to proper healing.

If you exercise regularly, you may think that you are appropriately challenging your body with the workouts you do. A common misconception of the layperson who works out and, unfortunately, even of some fitness professionals is that as long as you're doing *something*, you're helping yourself. This is not necessarily true regarding strength training. First, if you weight train and do only a few exercises, you could be adding to or creating muscle-imbalance issues. Second, if you never vary your workout or the exercises that you do, you will again be adding to or creating muscle imbalances. When Dennis, a forty-six-year-old client, first came to see me, he was so proud of the consistency of his workouts. Three times a week for two years, Dennis did the same weight-training exercises. I had to break the news to him that this workout had stopped benefiting him a long time ago.

Finally, if most or all of the exercises you do involve machines and sitting or lying fully supported at all times, you're never challenging your deeper stabilizing muscles, called your core. Thankfully, recent trends in fitness have begun to address this aspect of health. But a word of caution for you and your fitness trainer: for someone who has muscle imbalances and structural-alignment issues, doing core exercise training can reinforce compensation patterns.

Core Beliefs

A helpful way to convey the concept of our muscular arrangement is with the "ski suit analogy." In cold-weather skiing, you always dress in layers. You start with a light, thin T-shirt against the skin. Then you add a turtleneck over that. Next you may add a sweater to cover the turtleneck. And finally, you put on your thickest layer, your ski jacket. Your muscles are layered in a similar way. Your body has very small, intricate muscles that lie deep within you, called "core" muscles. The outer jacket might be the most expensive, most technologically advanced layer of clothing, but it still cannot do the job of the T-shirt. Like the thin T-shirt beneath all the other layers of clothing, the core muscles can't be seen, but they will be heard if they're not properly conditioned.

Your core is made up of the region around your hips, pelvis, and trunk. Most areas of the arms, the legs, the hands, and the feet are one and two layers deep. However, most people who exercise are exercising only the ski jacket. That is, they're exercising only the bigger, most superficial muscles that everyone sees. They essentially exercise for aesthetic reasons. Exercising this way is not wrong, but it is incomplete. When dealing with musculoskeletal pain, injuries, and rehabilitation, function must take priority over aesthetics.

The pelvis, more than any other structure in the body, has the greatest mechanical influence over the rest of the body. If the pelvis is off in its pitch from front to back, if it lists to one side or rotates left to right or right to left, it can alter the positioning of other parts of the body that are above and below it. This alteration can reach as far down as the feet and as far up as the head and the neck. The strongest and the largest sections of connective tissue in the body attach to the pelvis at the lower back, the abdominals, and the outer hips. And don't forget, this is where our center of gravity is located.

For someone challenged with a repetitive stress injury of the wrist or a knee problem, a question that might arise is, "What has the core got to do with my problem?" This is a good question, because there seems to be a more obvious relationship with back pain or hip pain when we discuss the core. The core equates to our center. All movements emanate from the core. For instance, if you are handwriting a letter at your desk for twenty minutes, you may experience "writer's cramp." This is when the small muscles in your hand become overworked. These working muscles are anchored on the wrist. Muscles that cross over the elbow joint dictate the position of the wrist. Muscles that cross over the shoulder joint control the elbow joint's position. And the muscles that cross over the shoulder joint are anchored to our core.

When alignment is good and the core is stable, the body is able to distribute more of the workload throughout the arm and the back to the core. The small muscles in the hands and the wrist are not designed to stabilize *and* perform hours of uninterrupted fine motor tasks. Here's a little demonstration to help you feel how simply changing your sitting posture can affect how you use the muscles in your forearm. Sit on a chair in front of your desk or dining table. In one hand, hold a tennis ball or even a rolled-up pair of socks. Rest your hands and wrists on your desk or dining table. Your hand should be on top of the ball, with the ball resting on the desk. Now slouch completely so that your back and shoulders are rounded and your head is forward (see figure 14). From this position, squeeze and release the tennis ball five to ten times, noting exactly where you feel the contraction and how strong it feels.

Shake out your hand, and rest for about twenty seconds. Then, sit up very straight so that your lower back has a little arc and your shoulders are back in line with your torso (see figure 15). Once again, place your hands on the table and squeeze and release the tennis ball five to ten times. Note where you feel the contraction this time and the strength of that contraction.

What typically happens in this demonstration is that while in the slumped

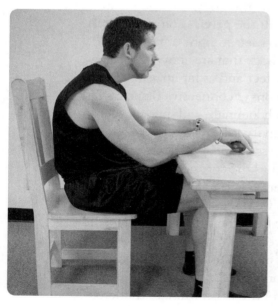

Figure 14
Slouching with tennis ball

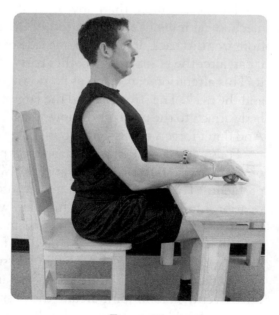

Figure 15
Sitting up straight with tennis ball

posture, you'll feel the contraction in a specific, concentrated region, usually in the forearm muscles facing the desk. The contraction feels strong in that region. With a more upright posture, you typically feel the contraction over a broader area, and the contraction is more diffuse. This is a demonstration of the body distributing the workload more efficiently. The advantage to doing this is to allow the small, intricate muscles of the hands and the wrists to occupy themselves with fine motor tasks, for which they are well equipped. It's when they're asked to pull double duty, to perform fine motor tasks *and* stabilize the involved body segment, that they become overworked. A constantly overworked muscle is not a happy muscle. If this overstress occurs repeatedly, the muscles' properties will actually begin to change. Metabolic by-products, which are the waste products produced by the muscles, gather within the muscle. Also, certain parts of the muscle become more like scar tissue (think beef jerky) and less like the smooth, soft fibers they should be. This creates a muscle that no longer functions the way it was designed to, negatively affecting the joints and the nerves in and around it.

Collecting the Data

As mentioned earlier, your proprioceptors (those sensitive structures in the muscles and the joints) are information gatherers that bring crucial data to your brain. Proprioceptors are one of three types of feedback mechanisms that your body has. The other two are part of the amazing radar system in your head: your eyes and your inner ear. The proprioceptors can be found in the muscles, the tendons, the joints, and the skin. They are sensitive to conditions like muscular tension and changes of length in muscles, as well as changes in joint position, pressure, and temperature.

Your vision is extremely important because it allows you to choose external points of reference. With your eyes, you constantly reference your relationship with the environment. Using your vision also allows you to find and focus on a fixed point when your balance has been disrupted.

All of your feedback mechanisms (your proprioceptors, eyes, and inner ear) may fool you into thinking that everything is okay with how your body is moving. This is because you have no point of reference other than yourself. If your feedback mechanisms don't feel as if anything unusual is going on, they'll continue to supply you with the same bad information that your body has adapted to. Often, what feels "right" is very wrong for the body.

The Villains We Don't Think About

When providing pain solutions for my clients, I often encounter a series of "villains" they blame for their complaints. Age is a popular evildoer, as is the individual's employer for bad working conditions, or the other driver who caused the accident that led to the injury, but let's look at some possible villains you might not have considered. As you read this book, consider the position your body is in right now. My guess is that you're either sitting down or lying down. If you're sitting, where are your hands? In front of you holding the book, right? Now take notice of where your head and shoulders are. Your head is down, with your shoulders rounded forward, along with your upper back. If you're lying down on your back and reading, how many pillows do you have behind you, pushing your head forward? And when your head is forward, think about what that does. It also causes your upper back to round forward, doesn't it? And your head and upper back cannot round forward without your shoulders doing the same. Do you remember when you were a kid and you studied or read lying on your stomach? You could rest on your elbows and read in front of you. Is that kind of movement of your hips and lower back a distant memory? It shouldn't be.

Let's go back to the sitting position. How many other things do you do sitting with your hands in front of you? You eat, drive, type, sew, cook, and write, just to name a few. Think about how many appliances in your life have made things "easier" for you by requiring less physical work on your part. The remote control for the television, the electric can opener, the dishwasher, power locks and windows on the car, automatic garage door openers, and on, and on, and on. Who are these innovations reducing the workload for? They're making sure that the guy who spends seven and a half hours of an eight-hour day in a chair in front of a computer or in a car seat doesn't have to move too much! The point is that as technology advances and our lifestyles become less physical, we must find a way to activate the muscles that are no longer used in the activities of daily life. We must introduce stimuli to our bodies that will counter the negative effects that our technologically advanced world places upon us. We live in a tunnel in regard to our physical movement. That tunnel is dictated by the lifestyles we have created for ourselves. We spend countless hours at home and at work, moving within a fraction of the range of motion that our bodies are capable of. We use the minimal amount of muscle activity that is available to us, and most of that activity comes from the larger, prime moving muscles. This means that the very important, deep stabilizing muscles are left unused. As the saying goes, use it or lose it. This lesson is learned the hard way if we injure ourselves taking groceries out of the car or while rushing across the street to beat traffic. We have stepped out of the tunnel that we've created, woefully unprepared. And when we leave this tunnel of daily living to "exercise," we step right in to another tunnel dictated by modern weight-training machines, cardiovascular-training machines, or 250 days a year of the same activity (tennis, golf, running, etc.).

Some of you might use your bodies all day long; in that case, the seven and a half hours of sitting doesn't apply to you. However, you must also consider the variety or lack thereof that your work requires. Just because you're moving every day doesn't mean that you're moving correctly. Most people who move frequently at work repeat a lot of the same movements, based on their job requirements. Therefore, a lot of movements may be performed, but many are the same movements. This leads to increased strength and efficiency in these movements, but often at the cost of their opposing movements. We must consider the "quality" of the movement versus the "quantity." So, if you move a lot each day, but have little variety in your movements, you're in the same tunnel as someone who gets on the stair machine every time she works out or a golfer who plays three to four times a week. We will get further into this concept of "quality" movement in the next chapter.

Aaron, the guy who sits for seven and a half hours a day, might argue that he leaves work and goes to the gym for ninety minutes every day. Then I would have to pose a similar question to him. "How much variety does your workout regime provide for your body?" He may benefit his cardiovascular system with aerobic exercise, but he may also do more overall damage to his musculoskeletal function with resistance (weight) training and not even know it. If you add a resistance (weights or gravity) regimen to an existing dysfunction in your musculoskeletal system, then you're reinforcing that dysfunction or developing additional compensatory dysfunctions. For example, let's say that one of your shoulders is lower than the other, and you're using a machine in which you press a weight over your head to work your shoulder muscles (often called a military press). The lever arm on the machine that you're pressing is even. Thus, the machine's designer has assumed that whoever uses it will have even shoulders. But, as we know, this isn't the case with you, so you have to put your hands on a lever that's even on both sides. The only way to do this is to compensate with the lower shoulder to make it even with the other shoulder. You do this by elevating or "shrugging" your lower shoulder. But when you do this, you engage a completely different muscle group that shouldn't be involved in this movement. At the same time, there will even be slight changes at the angles of your wrist, elbow, and shoulder joints as a result. Therefore, each and every time you perform this exercise, you reinforce the compensation that your body must make so that your hands are even on the machine handles. Your body adapts to the machine at the expense of compromised body mechanics.

Ultimately, the villain is not the other guy; it is the lifestyle you create to save time, reduce costs, and be more efficient. It's the equivalent of taking a wild animal that runs free, hunts for food, climbs, avoids its enemies, and so on, and locking it up in a zoo. In this life of confined movements, with limited energy expended for basic survival, an animal will pace the cage, bite the bars, and try to escape. The animal knows that this is not where it belongs or how it should live. But humans in industrialized nations don't display this sensible kind of behavior. We are all too content to opt for convenience and comfort, never realizing their negative impact on our health.

The "Healing Deficit"

Since our bodies are organic, the traumas we experience that don't kill us should heal. And for the chronic pain sufferer, the cuts, the bruises, the fractures, the sprains, and the strains do heal, but the pain doesn't go away. Now, it's not the cuts, the bruises, and so on, that are responsible for the pain. Instead, pain results from how these injuries have affected the body's mobility. A contributing factor to this pain relates to how the body was used prior to the accident or the trauma. Whatever the individual did wrong with his or her body before the accident could be interfering with the healing process weeks, months, and even years later. We stress this critical concept to many of our clients; most people have never considered it as a possibility.

Here's an example that I like to use in my clinic. For argument's sake, let's say that your job involves sitting at a desk. Now, imagine that you have a bad bruise on your knee. Your job requires that you get up and down from your chair twenty or thirty times a day. And every time you sit back down in your chair, you bang that bruised knee on your desk. The bruise will take a lot longer to heal in this scenario than it would if you just left it alone and allowed the body to heal itself. The same thing happens to people with neck, or shoulder, back, or hip problems that surface as a result of an accident. They aggravate their injuries every day, just on a much subtler level—but it happens more consistently, based on the ways they use their bodies. How people sit, stand, get up from the table, take a shower, get out of the car, and so on, doesn't seem to be a big deal, yet it can constantly impede the healing process. The cumulative effect of repetitive, improperly performed movements never gives the body a window of opportunity to adequately apply its healing capacities. I call this being in a state of "healing deficit": your body never reaches a point where it is no longer acting self-destructively. And if you think that bed rest or staying off your feet is the answer, think again. First of all, you have probably already tried this, and it didn't work. But more important, even if you start to feel better and begin to climb out of the healing deficit, without changing your improperly performed movements, you'll lose any progress you've made. Eventually, you'll be right back to the same point of the healing deficit. A simple analogy to clarify this would be someone with severe feline allergies. Let's say this person has spent a few hours in a room with several cats. This is a form of animal test that I approve of because no one gets hurt. Our subject will obviously have a strong allergic reaction to the cats. Once that reaction is present, it isn't likely to go away as long as the person is in the same room as the cats. Take the person out of the room, and within a few hours, he or she is back to normal, having recovered from the allergic reaction. Put the individual back into the same room with the cats, and the process is repeated. Take the person out of the room again, and allow him or her to recover. Bed rest is the equivalent of removing someone from the room to recover but then returning the person to the same cat-filled room.

6

Function First, Everything Else Follows

As I've mentioned, one of my key philosophies is to focus on the function of the individual's body, rather than attempting to treat or fix what hurts. The terms *function*, *functional*, and *functional exercise* have recently become commonplace in the health and fitness industries. The terms have been part of the physical therapy arena for at least ten years, but often without any clear agreement on exactly what they mean.

Most professionals will say that these terms are generally used to describe exercises or movements that relate to "real-world" situations or are "transferable," in that their benefits can be transferred to activities of life or sports. An exercise such as squatting is considered functional because it mimics movements that are used in getting up from and sitting down in a chair. The purpose of doing these types of exercises is to increase muscular strength and endurance for real-world activities. In the rehabilitation setting, functional exercises typically focus on the skills required for normal movement and independent living. For example, a person with knee surgery has to learn to walk properly again after years of having pain in the knee. Walking properly would include the position the foot must be in when the heel hits the ground and how the body weight must pass over the leg with the repaired knee. This cannot be achieved by rehabilitation that is done lying or sitting down.

In the athletic arena, functional exercises are more apt to apply to sport-specific skills. They also seek to strengthen and balance some of our more primal movement patterns that are foundations for sport-specific skills. An example of this type of exercise might be the lunge, which emphasizes independent balance requirements for both legs, while strengthening the legs in a functional movement. Athletes are often in scenarios while competing that require them to rapidly accelerate or change directions, using one leg to initiate the movement.

As part of the message of this book, we want to think in broader terms, using a higher set of standards, when we consider function. What do I mean by this? Well, if we return to the knee patient who must learn to walk properly again, "function" applies to the leg being rehabilitated. Typically, this would be the joints above and below the injured joint: the hip and the ankle of the injured leg. But true function should include the entire body, regardless of a specific area of injury. For a person to be functional, he or she must score high in the areas previously mentioned (in chapter 3) as assessable in the standing posture: muscle balance, mechanical efficiency, neuromuscular coordination, and kinesthetic awareness. If the individual scores high in these areas, then the body will move the way it was designed to move: efficiently, effectively, and with no undue stress on its parts. Moving functionally allows us to live more comfortable and productive lives.

Truly functional exercises employ more than one area or one joint in the body, even if certain parts of the body are used primarily for stabilization, while others perform most of the movement. On the other side of the coin are nonfunctional and dysfunctional exercises. Nonfunctional exercises often serve no purpose other than aesthetics and building muscle mass. Dysfunctional exercises promote dysfunctional movements and are potentially harmful. They can place inappropriate stress on the tendons, the bones, and the ligaments of the body. Such stresses leave these structures subject to breakdown and, ultimately, to injury. Common sense and an increased number of fitness professionals help to prevent most people from performing dysfunctional movements. Interestingly, however, when certain individuals do nonfunctional exercises, these become dysfunctional exercises. This scenario repeatedly occurs in health clubs and gyms across the globe. People believe they are lifting weights and doing resistance exercises for their health, but instead they end up injuring themselves. Most of the time, people aren't aware that they're hurting themselves by the way they perform exercises because the injuries don't occur acutely. Instead, their progressive onset can coincide with many other events in the individuals' lives.

Dysfunctional Exercise

Let's look at a very popular and common exercise, the bench press. This is a *nonfunctional exercise* that, for many people, is also a *dysfunctional* exercise. It's nonfunctional because the lifter is lying flat on his or her back to perform the exercise. Lying flat on your back is the most stable position you can be in. Therefore, the lifter has no real need to call upon any of the central stabilizing muscles to perform the lift. A major portion of the stabilization is provided by the effect of gravity on the lifter's body. Gravity holds the lifter's body to the bench that he or she is lying on. Then, if we look at the lift itself, it's a movement against resistance that no one is ever required to do in daily life. Even a person who does physical labor all day long wouldn't be in a position where he was lying on his back and pushing away repeatedly. The closest thing to a real-world application for this movement is the offensive lineman in football who puts his hands out in front of him to push away the oncoming defensive lineman. But even this technique cannot be accomplished without the offensive lineman planting his feet on the ground and having a strong base to push from. And if you think that because you use a sitting bench-press machine, you're doing a functional exercise, you're incorrect. It's essentially the same movement with just another fulcrum added. You are still stabilized by the machine.

This exercise becomes dysfunctional for an individual who already has strong and tight (short) muscles in the front chest and the shoulder muscles and is weak in the opposing muscles of the upper back and the shoulder blade region. This imbalance causes the shoulder blades to move away from the spine in the back, which, in turn, causes the shoulder's ball-and-socket joint to rotate down and in, leaving the entire shoulder girdle complex in a dysfunctional position. The dynamics of this joint have changed, causing the lifter to place continual stress on the tendons and the ligaments of the shoulder every time he or she does the bench-press exercise. This individual will usually end up with bouts of rotator cuff ailments, various shoulder/neck problems, or all of these. Depending on other structural issues (e.g., pelvic alignment), the symptoms may switch from one shoulder to the other. The usual course of self-treatment is to take time off from the exercise, swallow some ibuprofen, and/or use dumbbells that restrict the movement less. This certainly is not a way to solve the problem long term. In reality, the most basic intervention for this person would be to stretch out all of the anterior chest and shoulder muscles (pectorals major and minor, deltoids, latissimus dorsi, and biceps) and strengthen the muscles in the upper back (rhomboids, middle trapezius, extensor muscles of the thoracic back, and rotator cuff) to help place the shoulders in a more functional position.

Most of the exercises that people do in the gym are perfect examples of nonfunctional exercises. Another very familiar exercise is the leg-extension machine, which has a sitting bench and back support. The bench is high enough that your feet are off the ground, and a pad rests across the front of your ankles. From this position, you straighten your knee(s), lifting the pad that's across the ankles. This pad is connected to some type of resistance which is raised and lowered by your using the quadriceps (the front thigh muscles). Again, where in your day as a mom, a dad, a garbage man, or a computer programmer will you perform this motion? The closest movement I can identify with this exercise is the kicking motion of soccer players—and a kicking motion still requires synergistic movements at the hip and the ankle that the leg extension doesn't address.

The bench press and the leg extension are examples of many exercises that the fitness industry has adopted from the body-building community. The origin of these two exercises and others like them came from the need to overload and isolate specific muscles or muscle groups for the purpose of muscle hypertrophy or muscle growth. Other examples of similar exercises are the hamstring curl, the bicep curl, calf raises, and the tricep extension. Essentially, a nonfunctional exercise is any exercise that isolates a specific muscle or muscle group in a way that cannot be applied to life, work, rehabilitation, or sport. Does that mean we should do away with these exercises? I don't believe so. The use of these exercises has to be tied to the specific goals of the exerciser. If muscle hypertrophy is one of your goals, nonfunctional resistance exercises and machines can be a valuable part of your arsenal, but only *one* part of your arsenal. All of these exercises used on their own, without any stabilization training, muscle balancing, and three-dimensional movements, will leave you with significant structural weakness and problems with muscle coordination. Unfortunately, that is what happens to most exercisers. As a matter of fact, what many equipment manufacturers tout as a selling point has long-term detrimental effects for the user. The fact that a machine "supports your lower back" or keeps you completely stable deters from your ability to use those exact muscles when you are out of the gym and living your life. The only way to improve your physical being is by challenging it. Sitting on a recumbent stationary bike for twenty minutes may challenge your cardiovascular system and work your legs, but it does nothing to assist you with weaknesses around the mechanical center of your body. Nor does it allow your hip joints to move through a normal range of motion while you ride the bike. The "challenge" to your body should be relative to your current level of conditioning and function. Remember, there is never a one-size-fits-all exercise program. If you go to a gym and are given one of the "orientation" personal training sessions, be very careful. Typically, these are just a quick way to show you how to use a few machines so that you don't walk aimlessly around the gym. Unless the trainer has taken your health history and done some type of musculoskeletal assessment, you're getting the same orientation as everyone else in your demographic. If you really want to do things right and not waste time when doing resistance training, take a few training sessions to at least get you started. Research the qualifications of the staff, chat with various members to see if there is a personality match, and, most of all, clarify your goals and what you need from them.

Machines are not all bad, though. In their defense, machines are an excellent learning tool for the beginning exerciser. When a novice exerciser gets on a weight-training machine, he or she has fewer things to worry about when performing the movement than with free weights. This allows the novice to learn the new movement without expending physical and mental energy to stabilize the body while the primary movement is performed. The machine also guides the user through the movement to ensure that the appropriate muscles are being worked. Machines offer creative ways to manipulate the force of gravity and thereby challenge certain muscle groups with more variety than is possible with free weights, which purely oppose gravity.

Functional Exercises

So, what are some of the specific advantages of a functional exercise, and why is it important to you? First, let's reiterate that functional exercises and movements have real-world applications or are transferable to real-world tasks. Our real world involves movement in three-dimensional space. Real-world applications may be activities of daily living, work, or athletics. And for each person, they are different. Why? Because a new grandfather who wants to get stronger to lift his grandson, a college baseball player training in the off-season, and a forty-year-old mother recovering from a car accident will all wish to achieve different levels of function. In addition, each of these individuals will have strengths and weaknesses relative to his or her past physical history, and these strengths and weaknesses should be evaluated. If you're working with a personal trainer (or you plan to work with one), and the trainer has put you on a resistance-training program, ask how he or she decided which exercises to give you. The usual response will be that the trainer gave you a "well-rounded" or "balanced" workout to challenge every major muscle group. But if you challenge each muscle group equally in a "well-rounded" or "balanced" workout, then you *are* getting stronger, but you're maintaining the same muscle-imbalance ratios that you started with. This is why it's essential for your trainer to evaluate your posture prior to designing your exercise program. A postural evaluation can provide all the necessary information in a very usable and practical way within the gym or health-club setting.

The same argument applies to generic home exercises that are most often given by physical therapists and chiropractors. What good is doing back extensions on a machine or even on the floor if your body is not aligned first? If one hip is higher than the other and the muscles on that side of your back are shorter, aren't you just strengthening your back in the same dysfunctional position? The parts of your body that you wish to strengthen must first be in a functional position before you strengthen them. Again, this information is easily identified in the standing postural evaluation. For the health-care provider or the fitness professional whom you might work with, the information identified in the postural evaluation, combined with an appropriate knowledge of kinesiology and biomechanics, can readily predict what your body will do under dynamic conditions (i.e., movement).

So, where do you begin to gain function? For starters, becoming more functional is something that you, and only you, can do for yourself. Of course, it helps to get guidance from a knowledgeable professional, but the actual changes to your neuromuscular system occur from what you do and not from what someone else does to you. As mentioned earlier, the benefits of manual intervention performed by others on your body can be an integral part of the process, but without you driving the ship, long-term changes will not occur. Without these changes, you probably won't achieve the level of physical capability and the quality of life that you desire. If methods of passive intervention (medication, chiropractic, body work, acupuncture, etc.) are the only tools in your toolbox, there's no better time than right now to proactively change your body.

The next chapter will help you become a more functional person. You'll find exercises to perform that are based on who you are and what you do. The development of all the exercise programs was guided by specific principles from the Function First philosophy. These principles have been discussed throughout this book. You will select an exercise program based on your self-evaluation. It's okay to get help from someone else, but remember, you are the head coach of your team.

The exercises you'll perform are the building blocks for more advanced and challenging exercises. This is a necessary part of the reeducation of your body. You've heard the saying "You must walk before you run." Well, I like to take things back a step further than that. You must crawl before you walk. The exercises, first and foremost, will influence the segments of your body relative to one another. In other words, if we return to the blueprint of the human body in the standing position (figures 6 and 7), we can see that in order to achieve optimal alignment, the various segments of the body must sit in their appropriate places. If they don't, there is an alteration of body alignment, followed by an alteration of body mechanics that produces stress and the breakdown of affected areas. Where muscle tightness is present, this will increase; where there are inhibited and dormant muscles, those muscles will get weaker. Please note that figures 6 and 7 are not my interpretation of how the body should be aligned when standing. They are identical to any charts on the wall of a doctor's office or in an anatomy text, and that's because this is exactly how we should look when we stand.

If you seek to influence the alignment of your body segments in the direction of the blueprint, you must accept one very basic assumption: that the strategies your body uses for most of your fundamental movements and static postures are incorrect. The basis for this assumption is rooted in the principle that the alignment blueprint is the foundation for all of your movement patterns. And if your alignment isn't optimal, it will be very difficult for your movements to be optimal and pain-free. This, of course, brings us back to compensation. We don't want compensation, so the way we avoid it is by breaking the exercises down to a level where it's almost impossible for your body to compensate. This also happens to be a perfect level to begin the reeducation process for your muscles.

In the text "Motor Control: Issues and Trends" (1976), S. W. Keele, an expert in motor learning, developed an excellent example of how your body acquires new motor skills. In the case of most adults and people reading this book, it may be more appropriate to say motor *re-learning*. I have adapted his analogy so that you can easily associate it with your own experiences. If you look at the following chart, you can see how the act of driving a car with a stick shift can be represented at different stages of skill acquisition. Each movement has to happen, and they have to happen in this order for the driver to achieve the desired outcome of changing gears and moving the car. In this diagram you can see the heading for each action that's necessary to complete the shifting of gears (Accelerator Up, Clutch Down, etc.). If you try to move the shifter without pressing down on the clutch, you will damage the transmission. And if you try to put down the clutch without easing off the gas, the engine will rev too fast, overtaxing parts of your engine.

Down the left-hand side of the chart, you'll see the three progressions of practice. I'd like you to take a pencil and do something right now. If you don't want to write in your book (or if it's not your book), get a piece of scrap paper and write the numbers 1 through 7 in three rows. Label them just as they are in the book with the three types of practice (Early, Middle, and Late). You can reference your book for the headings over numbers 1 through 7 so that you don't have to write them all out.

Take your pencil and begin with the row labeled "Early Practice." Draw a circle around each of the seven numbers in that row. Next, go to the row labeled "Middle Practice" and draw one circle that includes the numbers 1 and 2. Next, draw another circle that includes the numbers 3, 4, and 5. Then, draw one more circle that includes 6 and 7. Finally, go to the row labeled "Late Practice" and draw one circle that includes all of the numbers from 1 through 7.

GEAR SHIFT ANALOGY

	Accelerator Up	Clutch Down	Shift Lever Forward	Shift Lever to Right	Shift Lever Forward	Clutch Up	Accelerator Down
Early Practice	1	2	3	4	5	6	7
Middle Practice	1	2	3	4	5	6	7
Late Practice	1	2	3	4	5	6	7

The purpose of circling each number in the "Early Practice" is that each one represents an individual task that must be learned for the driver to shift gears. In other words, each number is an entity in and of itself to the beginner. The driver cannot learn to drive the car until he or she is clear about what each step requires and how to perform it. That's why the steps must be considered individual components and be circled individually. Once the driver has mastered steps 1 through 7 in the "Early Practice" stage, he or she moves on to "Middle Practice." In "Middle Practice," we have circled the numbers in three groups. This is when our student begins "chunking" steps that must coincide with one another. Steps 1 and 2 are together because the driver can move the clutch and the accelerator at the same time. Steps 3, 4, and 5 are together because they all involve movement of the stick shift from the start position to placing it in gear. And, finally, 6 and 7 go together because they consist of flip-flopping the position of the clutch and the accelerator to begin moving the vehicle.

In "Late Practice," all of the steps are within one circle. This denotes a sequential series of movements that is represented within our nervous system as one piece of the pie of driving a car. With all of this practice, our driver is now probably shifting while she talks on her cell phone; drinks her double decaf, no-whip, sugar-free latté; and changes the radio station all at the same time. Imagine how complicated all of our movements would be if we never got out of the "Early Practice" stage of learning. Or, a more compelling question is, "What would happen if you didn't master each component in 'Early Practice' but then moved on to 'Middle Practice'?" You might be doing some of the steps correctly or all of them partly correctly, but not all of them completely correctly. And if no one is there to instruct you and give you feedback, you'd assume that you were doing everything right, even if you weren't. Therefore, you'd think that you were ready to move on to "Late Practice." So, you would then do everything sequentially and without having to think about the steps, but you have carried mistakes from "Early Practice" all the way through to the end of what you assume is a mastered task. Is this beginning to sound like it might apply toward your body as well? I hope so. Remember when I talked about the "baseline" the body sets for itself as normal? It is normal based on the body's own frame of reference and nothing else. The same holds true for our gear-shift analogy, unless feedback is provided by someone who has the proper experience and skill in driving a gear shift.

So, you may wonder, how do I teach this old dog new tricks? You do it by returning to the basic steps, the "Early Practice," so that you can provide your body with the appropriate stimuli for change. This is the beauty of the exercises in the next chapter. They will do just that.

The learning process can also be viewed in three phases. The first is the "cognitive" phase. This is the mental side of learning. During this phase, you will process the instructions or your options on how to perform a specific movement-related task. It may involve some visualization as well. Everything in the cognitive phase is done on an intellectual level, just as absorbing the information in these initial chapters has been. This is a very important first step, because if you aren't clear about your objective and what it takes to achieve it, you probably won't perform the movement correctly.

The second phase of learning is the "associative" phase. In this phase, the individual begins to learn a new movement task by associating it with one of the existing central motor programs in the motor system's database. For example, think about someone on ice skates for the first time. You've seen it. The person moves about as fast as rush hour traffic on the Los Angeles freeway. He or she merely shuffles and slides across the ice. This is not skating. Instead, the individual is trying to walk on ice wearing thin-bladed, unfamiliar shoes. The act of ice skating is similar to, but not the same as, walking, but because walking is one of our fundamental movement patterns, a novice reverts to it.

Another example might be a baseball player who decides to take up golf. When he first swings a golf club, it almost inevitably looks like a ballplayer swinging at a low pitch. He may step toward the ball, instead of keeping his feet still as he swings and may allow his front elbow to bend too much during the back swing. There are definite similarities in the two swings, particularly with the rotation of the torso and the use of the arms, so it would be natural, then, for a baseball-player-turned-golfer to associate some of the baseball techniques with the new skill of swinging a golf club.

The third phase is the "autonomic" phase of learning, where the movement task becomes automatic. When a movement becomes automatic, there is essentially no need for cognitive processing. When the ice hockey player steps onto the ice and must get the puck, his first thoughts are *not* "Push out and away with the left foot, then out and away with the right foot." Instead, he anticipates where the puck will end up because the skating aspect of his game is automatic, or second nature. The accomplished golfer doesn't go through all of the steps her coach gave her during the swing itself. Each movement has been integrated enough so that the smooth swing is automatic.

Clearly, the importance of going through every step of these learning processes is for you to understand how your body works. Armed with this kind of information, you now understand the relevance of doing the more basic exercises that I suggest, regardless of your current strength or fitness levels. In our clinic, a professional athlete may be on the floor next to a sixty-five-year-old grandmother who really never exercised much in her life, and they are both doing similar exercises. Everyone must function first.

7

Form Follows Function

I will now help you choose the best possible exercises for your specific structural characteristics and your unique station in life. Your station in life refers to the types of physical activities and movements that you perform most frequently during an ordinary day. For most of you, that will have some correlation with your occupation, but even if you don't work, you'll be able to identify with one of the six Forms that I'll outline in this chapter.

Unlike other books and videos that feature a one-size-fits-all program for back pain, one for neck pain, another for rotator cuff injuries, and so on, this book will provide tools that are much more specific to you. I call the different classifications *Forms* because of the well-known scientific premise that form follows function. What you'll observe in yourself and others is a reflection of the improper use, or function, of the musculoskeletal system.

The first thing you'll need to do is evaluate your structure. I want to keep this process easy, so the evaluation will focus on major postural distortions. Because there are many different possible combinations with the human body, you may not fit perfectly into one of the Forms I provide. Just choose the Form that best resembles yours. You can evaluate yourself alone with a mirror, or you can have photos taken of yourself from head to toe. Someone could also assist you. It's best to be dressed in as little as possible, to avoid any interference from the way clothing fits or hangs. You will want to do the evaluation barefoot. New shoes and insoles have a way of altering your stance, and old shoes can magnify existing problems.

If you use a partner or photos, please consider making a plumb line. It's very simple to do and can also provide an excellent reference point while you conduct your evaluation. It's nothing more than a weight hanging from a string. You can even use a fishing weight tied to some string (don't use fishing line because it will be too hard to see). An actual plumb bob from a hardware store doesn't cost more than a few dollars. The plumb line will represent the gravity line that is referenced in our blueprint. Hang the plumb line from the top of a doorjamb or the ceiling. The weight or the plumb bob at the bottom should hang about half an inch to an inch from the floor. Be sure that you're standing on a level floor, regardless of which way you choose to do the evaluation.

With some of the Forms we'll look at, the most important characteristics will relate to the side view of the body. With other Forms, the front or the back view will be the most important. And in some instances, you'll have the front view of one Form and the side view of another. Therefore, I don't want you to assume that you are one Form and immediately go to those exercises. Be sure to evaluate yourself from the front and the sides if you are alone. Evaluate from the front, the back, and the sides if you're using a partner. Don't worry, I'll explain later how to proceed if a partner is helping you.

There is also a "pecking order," if you will, when one observes postural alignment problems. Certain issues must be addressed before others because they have a greater overall disruption to normal movement patterns. What this means is that you may have to do the exercises for one Form for a few weeks and then move on to another Form, based on your combined alignment findings. You can find additional photo samples of the Forms at www.movementbydesign.com.

I'll present some of the more common ailments associated with each particular musculoskeletal Form. Of course, no alignment issue is guaranteed to have any of these symptoms, but the associated biomechanical compensations make these particular ailments easier to manifest in the body.

The Forms

Form 1

This Form's primary deviation is identified when the person is viewed from the side. If we refer back to our blueprint, the gravity line runs from the ankle bone through the knee; then through the hip, the lower back, and the shoulder; and finally ending behind the ear. Our Form 1 example shows a significant displacement of the hip joint ahead of the ankle, the knee, and the shoulder joints (see figure 16). The front of the body has a "bowing" appearance from the toes to the neck. This creates a need for the head to protrude forward to balance out the body. The weight of the head counters the weight of the upper body, which is going backward. The upper body must go backward to counter the shift of body weight forward around the hips. With the hips forward like this, very often the knees will hyperextend. Here is a perfect example of the human body's need to balance its center of gravity (COG) over its base of support, the feet. In other words, if you have a zig, you must have a zag. The COG is balanced, but the body is contorted to do so. Therefore, balancing the COG over the base of support does not necessarily correlate with functional alignment (although they can).

Whenever the upper back rounds, the shoulder blades move away from the spine and the chest compresses. This causes the ball and socket of the shoulder joint to round inwardly. If the head were to follow the upper spine at this point, the person would fall backward, thus the need for the head to move forward.

This postural alignment is reflective of an individual who lacks structural strength through the body's central core. Essentially, this person is simply resting on the ligaments in the front of the hips. The individual uses very little muscular strength to maintain their alignment. Although this particular scenario requires less energy expenditure than optimal alignment does, the tradeoff biomechanically isn't worth it. The stresses placed on the body are too much and will ultimately lead to the tissue damage and pain that were discussed at length in earlier chapters. Optimal alignment displays the most advantageous distribution of work from muscular contractions, coupled with the built-in stability of the shapes of the joints and the passive tension created by tendons and ligaments. Form 1 places entirely too much responsibility on the passive tension of tendons and ligaments.

Major areas of stress for the Form 1 person will be the neck and the upper back, the lower back, and the knees. Muscularly, this person will have poor development of the buttocks muscles (gluteus maximus) and weakness in the hip flexor muscles. The muscles of

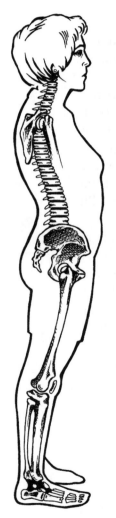

Figure 16
Form 1

the upper chest and the shoulders will be tight. The muscles in the back of the neck will also be tight. The muscles in the middle back will be lengthened and weak. Often, the person with the Form 1 alignment also has well-developed muscles on the back of the thighs (hamstrings) to compensate for the buttocks muscles.

Although a major characteristic of the Form 1 person is weakness through the body's core, it doesn't necessarily mean that this person is sedentary. While some sedentary people are representative of this Form, I also find plenty of active and athletic people.

Even though the Form 1 individual's hips are out in front when the person is standing, the structural weakness associated with this creates just the opposite effect when he or she sits. This person lacks the strength to maintain good alignment in the sitting position. While sitting, the Form 1 individual has a tendency to sit more on the lower part of the buttocks and the upper thighs. This causes the curve in the lower back to reverse directions, pushing the head and the shoulders even farther forward. For the Form 1 person who does detailed work with the hands, such as with computers or assembly, there is a high risk of upper-extremity, repetitive stress–type injuries, due to the change in dynamics of the shoulder girdle. This places greater overall stress on the soft tissue (muscles, tendons, and ligaments) of the upper body.

The reasonably active Form 1 person may often end up with problems away from the core of the body, due to the lack of core stability. This might include ankle, knee, and hip problems or shoulder and elbow problems for tennis or volleyball players and weight lifters. Lower-back pain may also be an issue when the person sits or stands too long. Changing position from sitting to standing can often provide temporary relief.

Form 2

Form 2 is also best identified by using the side view (figure 17). If we begin the observation at the feet, we can see that the angle of the ankle is changed due to the slight bend or flexion in the knee. This person often has flattened arches and stands with most of the body weight on the heels. From the side view, the overall flexion of the spine is also apparent. Instead of the spine presenting a

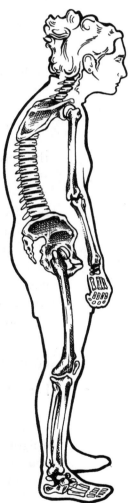

Figure 17
Form 2

nice, soft "S" curve, as it does in the blueprint, it has more of a "C" shape. This is highly correlated with the pelvis tipping backward. The landmarks on the back of the pelvis are lower than the landmarks on the front of the pelvis. If we imagined the pelvis as a bowl, when it is neutral the contents of the bowl will rest undisturbed. In Form 2, the contents of the bowl are spilling toward the back of the body. As the pelvis tips backward, the curve in the lower back is flattened. Although our gravity line runs closer to the hip joint in Form 2 than it did in Form 1, the head still protrudes forward. Again, the weight of the head is attempting to offset the body weight behind the gravity line.

Flexion begets flexion. If the lower spine is in flexion, the upper spine will follow the lower spine's lead and flex more. As we saw in Form 1, flexion of the upper spine again causes the shoulder blades to move away from their home close to the spine, rounding the shoulders forward.

This postural alignment is also a reflection of noticeable muscle weaknesses, along with the imbalances. The muscles that rotate the pelvis posteriorly, or backward, are stiffer and/or stronger than the muscles that rotate the pelvis anteriorly, or forward. The abdominals, the gluteals, and the hamstrings rotate the pelvis posteriorly. The hip flexor muscles and the muscles that extend the lower back rotate the pelvis anteriorly. This person will also be very weak in the muscles that extend the upper back, which is evident in the rounding (and, therefore, the prolonged lengthening) of these muscles.

Common ailments associated with this kind of postural alignment include sacroiliac joint (SI) pain, sciatica, bunions, plantar faciitis, upper-back and neck pain, temporomandibular joint (TMJ) problems, headaches, and repetitive motion injuries of the arms, the wrists, and the hands. The Form 2 individual may also regularly complain of excessive fatigue and weakness.

Form 3

Form 3 is the first Form that we'll evaluate from the front view. We can, however, also use the side view with Form 3 to confirm the pelvic tilt here. If you use the plumb line for the front view, remember that the plumb bob or the weight should always be centered between the feet. Don't try to line it up with your nose or your belly button. These parts of your body can move around as you stand, but the feet stay fixed once you put them where you want.

If we begin at the feet again, you'll see that the feet turn out at a 30-degree, or more, angle (figure 18). The feet should either be straight ahead or slightly toed out to about 10 degrees when in a functional position. Turning the feet out often reflects a rotation occurring at the hips and has very little to do with the feet. The feet just indicate what's happening higher up the chain. If you travel up from the feet to the knees, you'll see that the knees also point outward. Imagine that the fronts of your kneecaps are headlights on a car. If that car were traveling down the road, the headlights would shine off toward the sides of the road and not straight down the road in the direction the car is traveling. This outward rotation of both the feet and the knees comes from tightness in the muscles that rotate the hip out and weakness of muscles that rotate the hip in.

When we look at the front view of the arms in Form 3, we see that both the shoulders and the forearms rotate inwardly, or pronate. This is evident by the fact that we can see most of, or all of, the backs of this person's hands. The shoulders being rotated in on the Form 3 individual are different from the rounded shoulders in Forms 1 and 2. In Form 3, the upper back doesn't round, and the shoulder blades don't necessarily move away from the spine, as they do in Forms 1 and 2. Instead, the ball of the upper arm bone (humerus) turns inward within the socket of the shoulder blade (scapula).

Next, look at the Form 3 individual from the side view to confirm the front-to-back rotation, or "pitch," of the pelvis. The Form 3 person has an anterior or forward tilt to the pelvis (figure 19). This pelvis rotation places the major landmarks on the back of the pelvis higher than the landmarks on the front of the pelvis. If we again use the analogy of the pelvis as a bowl, the bowl would be spilling its contents toward the front of the body. This is often reflected by a protruding abdominal area and/or prominent buttocks.

The anterior rotation of the pelvis correlates with tightness in the hip flexor muscles and the lower back muscles.

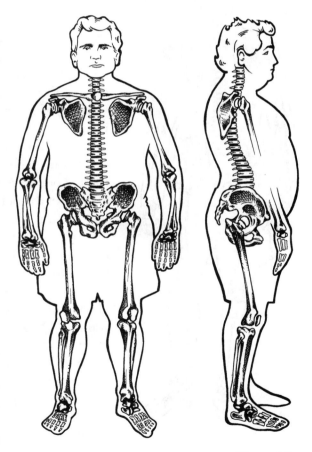

Figure 18
Form 3

Figure 19
Form 3 side view

Weakness in the antagonist, or opposing, muscles to the hip flexor muscles is also present. The antagonists include the gluteals (buttocks), the hamstrings, and the abdominals.

Common ailments associated with this kind of postural alignment include lower-back pain, spondylosis and spondylolesthesis, hip joint pain, groin strains, tight hamstrings, and rotator cuff problems. Form 3 individuals often refer to themselves as being "tight" and lacking overall flexibility.

Form 4

Once again, we'll view this individual from the front. The Form 4 person has characteristics that typically develop after a year or more of a dysfunction or during an acute spasm in the lower back. Interestingly, we don't often see this Form clinically until weeks or months after the initial event that affected the body, but that doesn't mean that it can't happen during that time period. So, if you identify with the characteristics of Form 4, then follow the appropriate exercises regardless of any time frame you associate with it.

As with the other Forms, let's start at the feet and work our way up. The Form 4 individual usually has only one foot rotated out more than the other (figure 20). The same knee and hip of the outwardly rotated leg will also rotate out. One leg may, in effect, appear turned out relative to the other one. The height of the pelvis on this same side will be higher than on the other side, so the pelvis slopes away from the side of the outwardly rotated leg.

One way to see this alignment is to put your hands on top of your hip bones, as if you were standing with your hands on your hips. You should notice that one side is higher than the other. Another clue is when you look at the skin folds that make up your waistline. On the high hip side, you'll see a higher crease along your side in the area of the waist.

Continuing up the body, we'll stay with the same side that has presented all of the structural issues thus far. The shoulder on this side has dropped or is lower than on the other side. This can be determined by viewing the heights of the shoulders as you look in the mirror. In addition, there

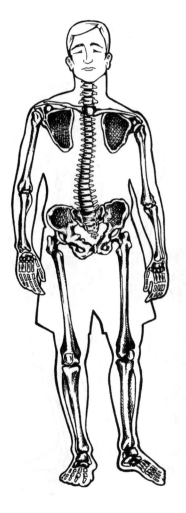

Figure 20
Form 4

appears to be more "space" between the lower shoulder and the neck that is not evident on the normal shoulder. Men with this problem often have to get their suits tailored to cover up this discrepancy. The sleeve lengths will have to be adjusted, and sometimes padding will be placed in the area of the lower shoulder to make the shoulders appear even.

The appearance of more "space" between the neck and the shoulder is a result of the shoulder being lower and the head leaning away from this shoulder. The tilting of the head makes sense if we refer back to our earlier discussion of the head acting as our radar system. The mechanisms in our ears and eyes seek to keep the body upright. If the head followed the dropped shoulder, it would end up resting on an angle. We would then view our world diagonally, and our brains don't process that well. Therefore, the head seeks to counter the dropped shoulder and center the body by bringing itself back toward the middle and away from the side that's leaning.

The body of the Form 4 person appears to be compressed on the side of the high hip and the lower shoulder, and that's essentially what's happening. The muscles have tightened, drawing the top and the bottom halves together. The muscles in the lower back and the buttocks that influence the hip joint have also tightened, causing the hip to rotate out.

This happens to someone who has a higher hip over a period of time because the body adapts to this posture. In contrast, a person whose pelvis is elevated on one side for a short period of time will often have a high shoulder on the same side as the high hip, as the body initially leans away from the higher hip.

With a back spasm, the pull will be so strong and abrupt the body has to drop the shoulder and lean the head away. Remember, the spasm is quite often the body's protective mechanism to prevent further injury, so an individual with a back spasm will unconsciously give in to the spasm to avoid increased pain and perhaps greater injury.

Muscularly, Form 4 has one-sided tightness of the lower-back muscles on the side of the high hip, as well as of the deep hip flexor muscle (iliopsoas). Muscles of the shoulder girdle will be stretched out and weak. Muscles on the side of the neck opposite the low shoulder may also be tight.

Form 4 is almost always associated with some form of lower-back pain. In addition, there is sometimes neck pain and pain that runs into the shoulder blade. The hip on the high side may also become arthritic and degenerative. If this posture has been assumed for many years, the Form 4 individual might have countless other symptoms, due to the havoc the posture wreaks on normal movement.

Form 5

The characteristics seen in Form 5 are not what most people think of when they consider posture. The layperson typically assesses other people's posture by viewing them from the side. Most health and fitness professionals view from the side, the front, and the back. But very few people, professionals and nonprofessionals alike, consider the view from above. Yes, from above. No, we don't stand on top of someone and look down, but that's the vantage point you have to imagine viewing the body from. The view from above provides us with a view of rotations. Some of my clients use the term *twisted* to describe their condition. Rotations can be seen at the foot, the knee, the hip, the pelvis, the torso, the shoulder, the forearm, the neck, and the head. For our purposes, and what is typically most significant, is rotation of the pelvis and the trunk.

If you're evaluating yourself, use a mirror. Standing in front of a mirror that allows you to view your hips and shoulders will best display rotations. If you can, stand only about two to three feet from the mirror, and directly face it. While facing straight ahead, close your eyes for about five seconds. Then place your index fingers on the two front "points" of your hips. In anatomical terms these points are called your anterior superior iliac spines, but all you need to know is that they are the most prominent front part of your pelvic bones. Once you've placed your fingers on those points, open your eyes and immediately look down at your fingers. Is one finger closer than the other to the mirror? If so, your pelvis is rotated.

Now look at your shoulders and upper body in the mirror. Is one shoulder closer to the mirror than the other? This part gets a little trickier because it's possible to have just the shoulder itself rotated forward and not the rest of the torso. To be sure that it's not just the shoulder, look at the chest and the shoulders together. Figure 21 is an example of a person with a rotation in both the pelvis and the torso, when viewed from the front. Figure 22 shows what the rotation would look like when viewed from the side.

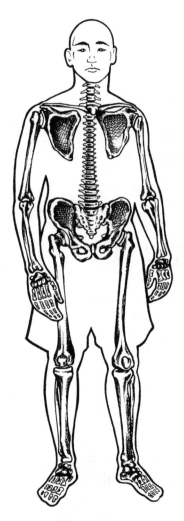

Figure 21
Form 5

One other area on your body to check is your knees from the side view. If you stand with one knee bent even slightly more than the other is, this could be a factor. Typically, the side of the body with the bent knee will be the side that rotates forward. If this is the case, you'll still have to address the learned rotational component of your pelvis and torso, because if you weren't aware of standing with one knee bent, then you've probably been standing that way for a long time. And straightening your knee alone won't remove the adapted rotations in your pelvis and torso.

It's possible to have only the pelvis or the torso rotated forward. It's also very common to have both the shoulder and the pelvis rotated at the same time. The problem with any of these three scenarios is that the eyes are looking ahead, making the body feel straight even though it is twisted. A safe assumption is that somewhere between the feet and the eyes, the body has twisted itself in one direction and then corrected back toward the other direction to keep the eyes pointing straight ahead.

Form 5 is one of the most detrimental Forms to the body. A rotated body conflicts more with our fundamental movements than do the other Forms. Consider the basic act of walking. Walking essentially occurs in a straight and forward plane of movement. Certain minor rotations occur at different parts of the body, but the overall movement is described as linear. Think of the stress placed on your body if your eyes and your feet direct your body straight to the north, but your pelvis and torso face northwest.

In addition, there is your body's need to rotate during daily and recreational activities. Consider a motion like getting out of a car. You certainly have to turn your body to do that. It requires a rotation of your hips and your upper body so that they can line up with your legs to lift you out of the car. Perhaps you're thinking that if you're already rotated, getting out of the car should be easier! And if you're rotated in the direction that you turn to get out of the car, you're correct. What happens to your body, though, when you get back into the car? Your body is biased toward movement in one direction. Therefore, you have to move your muscles and bones from a mechanically disadvantaged position to get back into the car. This requires more work and produces greater overall stress on the joints and the soft tissue.

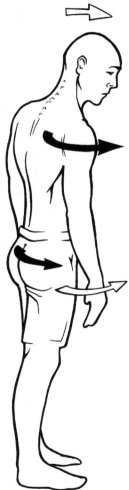

Figure 22
Form 5 rotation

A golfer might be the most obvious example of how damaging this Form is to the body. The golf swing is preceded by a back swing. If the golfer's body is biased in the direction of the golf swing, she will never be able to achieve a full back swing. She will then be limited in how far and how accurately she can hit the ball because the back swing must provide the necessary "coiling" of the muscles used in the swing. Another golfer's body might be biased in the direction of the back swing. This golfer may be able to get the club head way back before the swing, but he can't get his hips around to turn properly into the swing. This golfer probably slices the ball a lot because he can't get the club head around in time to transfer his weight and get the club's face directly on the ball.

Form 5 is caused by imbalances of the muscles that run from the hips to the neck. Very often it results from a one-sided involvement of the muscles that rotate the hips and the torso. It is likely to involve the oblique abdominals and perhaps one side of the erector muscles that run up and down the spine. This one-sidedness can be due to the body avoiding pain now or at some time in the past or can result from a repetitive pattern of working, as with a dentist who always sits on the same side of his patients and turns the same way while working on them. As with the other Forms, the individual probably wasn't aware that his or her body was "twisted." Once again, the body has set a baseline for what it perceives as normal.

The Form 5 person is more susceptible to hip joint pain and degeneration because the ball and socket don't line up properly, due to the rotated pelvis. Form 5 is also prone to lower-back pain and neck pain. The neck pain is often one-sided, due to the body's correction for the twisting below.

Form 6

We return to a side view evaluation for Form 6. When describing Form 6 to my clientele, I like to use the term *zig zag*. This Form is a clear case of an individual shifting one segment of the body in response to a shift in another. In order to keep the body balanced over the feet (and to avoid toppling over), this is a necessary adjustment. It usually begins with the pelvis and works its way up the spine to the head. At first glance, Form 6 can be confused with Form 1. Both of these Forms have issues related to the pelvis and corresponding changes in the curvature of the thoracic (upper) back.

If you recall in Form 1, as we viewed it from the side, the pelvis was displaced in front of our plumb line. The axis of the hip joint didn't line up with the plumb line. As a result, the upper back swayed backward to offset the forward movement of the pelvis. In Form 6, the rationale is the same, but the reasons are different.

As you view Form 6 from the side, begin at the feet, as we do with all of the other Forms (see figure 23). As we move up the body from the feet, the plumb line intersects the weight-bearing joints of the lower body (ankle, knee, and hip) reasonably well. So, unlike Form 1, where the hip joint was out in front of the line, in Form 6 the line runs through or almost through the hip joint. In Form 6, the crux of the problem lies with the forward tilt of the pelvis. If you remember our analogy in Form 3 of the pelvis as a bowl, we can apply that here. As with Form 3, the pelvis is pitched forward, or the bowl is spilling its contents on this person's toes. The critical identifying landmarks on the back of the pelvis are much higher than are the landmarks on the front. In Form 3, this was associated with a protruding abdomen and high, prominent buttocks. In Form 6, there still will be a protruding abdomen, but the buttocks won't be nearly as prominent.

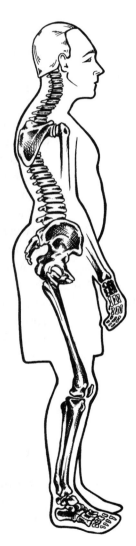

As we continue toward the head, you'll see that a significant amount of middle and upper torso is behind the line. This is the upper body's "zag" to the pelvic area's "zig." To again clarify the difference between Form 1 and Form 6, in the latter the angles of the curves in the lower back and the upper back are much more acute. By comparison, the curves in Form 1 are elongated and drawn out.

With this abrupt angle change in the upper back, the shoulders must round forward to bring the weight of the arms back in front of the gravity line. The head must also come forward to assist the person in re-centering the body over the feet. This is also the only way the person can reorientate his or her eyes with the horizon. If the individual didn't make this correction, the head would sit behind the shoulders, and the person would be staring at the sky while walking.

The characteristics of Form 6 often rear their ugly heads in adolescence. They may be found in taller children, who try not to stand out among their peers or in large-breasted teenage girls who attempt to hide their size. Left uncorrected, the abrupt curves we've identified in Form 6 will worsen with age. To all of you parents out there, the longer that any postural distortion is left unaddressed, the

Figure 23
Form 6

more the rest of the body tissue adapts to these distortions. With this goes an increased opportunity for pain to develop. The longer the postural faults are present, the more time and effort are required to correct it. Yelling at little Johnny to "Stand up straight" or telling young Suzy to "Hold your shoulders back" is never enough. In fact, it's only a drop in the bucket toward what needs to be done. Remember, for your own sake and the sake of your children, that our postural alignment is based on mechanics and reflexes. We can think, "Stand up straight," and we'll do it while we think about it, but as soon as our attention is drawn elsewhere, our bodies will return to the position they are accustomed to and are strong enough to maintain. I bring up this point about children with Form 6 because, in my experience, it seems to be most prevalent with adolescents. Yet the argument is the same for any of the Forms listed in this book. If your son or daughter is experiencing aches and pains, postural faults are probably the main reason.

Form 6 results from weakness in the abdominal and the gluteal muscles. The hip flexors are the antagonists to these muscles. The hip flexors will be tight and stiff, as will the lower-back muscles. In addition, the deeper muscles of the upper back will be lengthened and weak. The more superficial muscles between the shoulder blades will also be lengthened and weak. The antagonist muscles that are used to pull the shoulders forward are the chest and the biceps.

Middle-aged adults and older people who have had these structural issues for a long time will be prone to developing degeneration between the vertebral joints of the spine. This is due to a "wedging" that occurs between the front bodies of the vertebrae because of the sharp curves in the vertebral column. Therefore, lower- and upper-back pain is highly correlated with Form 6. Neck pain often occurs as well, due to the head position. Upper-extremity, repetitive-motion injuries are also common, as the dynamics of the upper body change due to the dysfunctional shoulder and head position.

Lifestyle and Occupation Classifications

Determining which of the six major Forms most resembles your posture is just the beginning. I want to help you take your self-diagnosis a step further and get even more specific. Instead of doing exercises merely to improve your looks, I want your exercises to also relate to what you do. If you are like most people, your occupation, your station in life, or even your former occupation, if retired, occupies half of your waking hours. You need some defense. And, as the sports analysts often say, the best defense is a good offense. I want you to go on the offensive with your exercise program. Provide your body with what it needs to neutralize the effects of your daily environment. Read the following descriptions of the occupations and the lifestyle categories. Few people will fit 100 percent of the time into a classification, but find the one that best describes how you spend most of your time. If it is split 50-50, then maybe you'll do two exercise programs on alternate days. Read on to find out where you fit best.

Category 1: Physical Workers

If you fall into this category, you couldn't do your job if your body broke down. Your body must physically respond to the tasks at hand. These can include lifting, carrying, loading, digging, climbing, bending, crawling, and the like. Physical strength and endurance are required to perform your job. Some examples of physical workers include

Labor/construction

Hospital orderlies

Warehouse workers

Delivery personnel

Landscapers

Category 2: Dexterity Workers

A dexterity worker must do a lot of fine motor skills with the hands. If you had your hand or wrist in a cast, it would be almost impossible for you to perform your job. The motions that you do are often very similar and repetitive. In order to perform these fine motor skills with your hands, the rest of your body is typically held in a static position while your eyes observe what you do. Some examples of dexterity workers include

Computer users

Laboratory workers

Assemblers

Dental hygienists

Hairdressers

Category 3: Multitaskers

If you don't fall into Category 1 or 2, you'll fall into the multitasking category. Your job or lifestyle may require many different tasks throughout the day, some of which include Categories 1 and 2. It will also probably involve getting into and out of the car, working in several or many different environments, and occasionally assuming awkward postures. Some examples of multitaskers include

Stay-at-home moms/dads

Postal workers

Restaurant/hospitality workers

Outside sales

Retail sales

At this point, you have two methods of identifying yourself for the purpose of choosing the right functional exercise program. You may even have three because through your postural evaluation, you realized that you have the characteristics of more than one of the Forms presented. That's okay because as we move on to the next chapter, the exercises for all the Forms and the Categories will be laid out for you, along with ample instructions.

Now that you've identified where you are in the world of Function First, it's time to take action. I hope that you performed a careful, thorough evaluation and even sought some help. Your intervention (the exercises) will be only as good as your evaluation. Remember, the exercises are designed to address specific structural imbalances. Apply the wrong exercises to your body, and you aren't likely to get any value from them. Worse yet, they might even add to your dysfunction. So, if you're not sure whether you did a good job with your evaluation, here's a chance to go back and double-check your initial view.

On my Web site are additional photos of individuals who represent examples of the 6 Forms (www.movementbydesign.com). In addition, the site contains other information to help you maximize your experience with the exercises and the advice in this book.

Once you're completely confident that you've identified the Form(s) that most resembles your structure, pair that up with the Category that best describes the bulk of your daily activities. Then, simply cross-reference the exercise program listed for that combination. For example, if you are Form 3 and Category 2, you'll use Exercise Program 3.2.

If you've identified yourself as fitting the description for more than one

Form, there's a progression to follow. This is because you must address certain deviations before others, based on the body's response to these specific deviations. The only two Forms that you can combine with any of the others are Form 4 and Form 5. Forms 1, 2, 3, and 6 cannot be combined with one another.

The rules for combining are as follows:

1. Form 5 is always the first Form that must be addressed. Exercises for Form 5 must be completed daily for ten to fourteen days before you move on to the exercises for the other involved Form(s). For example, if you identified yourself with the characteristics of Form 5 and Form 1, you must do the exercises assigned to Form 5 for ten to fourteen days before you move on to the exercises for Form 1.

2. Form 4 is always the first one addressed *except* when combined with Form 5. If you pair Forms 4 and 5 together or with another Form, Form 5 is always the first exercise program, as stated in Rule 1. The exercises for Form 4 are done for ten to fourteen days. The exercises for any other Forms will then follow the completed series for Form 4. If Form 4 is combined with either Forms 1, 2, 3, or 6, the exercises for Form 4 are done first for ten to fourteen days. Those exercises are then followed by the assigned exercises for the other Form.

The exercises are placed in an order that's critical to their success. Essentially, one exercise prepares the body for the next. I'm of the opinion that all exercise regimens should follow a logical sequence. This aspect of designing exercise programs is often overlooked by most fitness professionals and therapists. What good is it to have the seven numbers that make up someone's phone number if they aren't in the order that will cause that person's phone to ring? A logical progression is as applicable for a gym workout as it is for any corrective or therapeutic exercise program. Have you ever gone to the gym and structured your workout around which machines or weights were available? If you did, it was just to get the exercise done and not waste time. It wasn't to maximize the benefit of your workout, right? Or have you ever been given a handout by a therapist or a doctor with multiple exercises on it, after that individual had just circled a few of them? Are you supposed to do the exercises in the order they occur on the sheet? If so, the assumption is that the sheet was designed with a logical progression in mind. On the other hand, maybe the sheet was designed by grouping the exercises according to their level of difficulty or according to the apparatus (e. g., physioballs or tubing) involved. From the sheets our clients have brought to us, I can't decipher any particular method to the madness, other than the types of apparatus used.

Every kind of exercise has three components it: (1) biomechanical, (2) physiological, and (3) neurological. This is as true for running as it is for your first stretch to the ceiling when you get out of bed in the morning. The analogy of an automobile can be helpful here. The biomechanical or the mechanical component, as it relates to a car, would be the movement of the car itself. This applies to the weight of the car's body over the chassis, how the wheels turn, or how the shocks absorb bumps. The physiological component would be the engine, the fuel that runs the engine, and the oil that keeps the parts running smoothly. The neurological component would be the electrical components and, in today's cars, the microcomputers. These components send signals to all of the other parts to make things happen. How effective is a brand-new car if you don't have the key to turn on the ignition?

I emphasize these points because the exercises you'll do may appear quite remedial at first glance. This could not be further from the truth. Nearly every exercise has many more things occurring within it than may be apparent to the untrained eye. A great deal of thought has gone into each exercise and how it relates to the Form it addresses and the lifestyle that goes with it. Take full advantage of the sequencing of these exercises and resist the temptation to jump around in the sequence. Many people in our clinic ask if they can do all of the lying-down exercises together, all of the wall exercises together, all of the standing exercises together, and so forth, and so on. The answer is "no." That would disrupt the sequence. It also reduces the opportunity for you to assess the impact of each exercise as you transition from one position to the next. Life is about movement, so enjoy the process.

This brings me to another important point. While working with my clientele, I often ask them, "Where do you feel this?" during an exercise. All too often, their response is, "It doesn't hurt anywhere." Well, that's not really what I'm asking. What I want is a full-body self-assessment of muscle work, stretch, relaxation, pain, and so on. But instead, what I gain from this kind of response is two insights: the first, and probably the more important, is that any inventory this client has ever taken on his body relates to the level of pain. He has no connection with his body other than whether it hurts or how much it hurts. Remember our discussion about proprioception (body awareness)? This gentleman has none. He tunes out his connection to his body to avoid interpreting more pain. The second insight relates to his past experience with any therapy he has undertaken. He assumes that pain is a major part of the therapeutic process and that he should expect it. I beg to differ.

You should not expect pain when doing these exercises. Remember, the ultimate goal of improving your functional alignment is to provide your body with an optimal environment in which to heal. By doing so, you remove the negative stimulus or stimuli that create a pain response in your body on a regular basis. If this is clearly the goal, then reproducing your pain would be contrary to that. Let me reemphasize that: these exercises should not reproduce your pain. If an exercise does reproduce your pain, you will have to eliminate it or modify it if you can.

Let me also be clear that there's a distinction between reproducing your pain and experiencing discomfort from doing exercises that you've never done before. We're all familiar with the muscle soreness that occurs from stressing (exercising) a muscle we haven't stressed in a long time. This may occur, even with exercises that look simple. You may also stretch some tight muscles that haven't had their length disturbed in some time. A good rule of thumb to follow is that a stretch should never be so aggressive or intense that it's painful. Stretching a muscle to this extent will be counterproductive. You'll elicit a built-in defense mechanism that will cause the muscle to recoil immediately when you release the stretch. Even worse, the recoil is likely to shorten the muscle more than it was prior to the aggressive stretch. Mild discomfort is okay, but never painful stretching.

You will also do exercises that require you to contract and shorten muscles as part of the strengthening element of your program. These exercises require you to use only 50 to 60 percent of what your perceived maximum would be. One of the biggest mistakes people make with exercises designed to reeducate the body is to push or pull too hard. When you're trying to influence your neuromuscular system, harder is not better. As a matter of fact, it can be counterproductive. The best way to influence this system is through more subtle movements, rather than by exerting the effort that most people who exercise are familiar with. Remember, these aren't exercises for rippled abdominals or bulging biceps. Instead, they will influence the way the body's parts cooperate with one another.

There are two main reasons why you shouldn't work too hard (more than 50 to 60 percent). The first is to avoid using the same old strategies that your body has always used to produce any movement that's similar to the exercise at hand. For example, if you're doing an exercise with your arms and your tendency is to shrug your shoulders to stabilize yourself, that's what you'll do. Stabilizing yourself this way is inappropriate, but you're unable to recognize this error because you're concentrating more on the outcome of the exercise than on how to do it. In other words, you're thinking, "My arm has to go from here to there this many times, come hell or high water." We must back off from that all-out effort and think about how the arm got from here to there, *not* that the arm did manage to do so. This emphasizes the route the body uses, versus the final destination. And in the initial phases of the motor-learning process, the route is much more important.

The second critical reason is that when we push or pull too hard, we actually recruit the wrong muscle fibers to use. Not all of the fibers in your muscles are the same, and muscles will have different ratios of the varying muscle-fiber types. To avoid a physiology lesson here, let's look at how this applies to your goals in simple terms. If you push and pull too hard, you end up using the big, major muscles that are mostly responsible for gross motor movements. Gross motor movements are actions like walking, getting out of a chair, or lifting a bag of groceries. The body creates momentum with these muscles, but that isn't the purpose of the exercises. Because every muscle in the body has a specific function, we want to make sure that the muscle groups you target with these exercises give the "wake up call" to those hibernating muscles.

Resting between sets of exercises is also required. This isn't the same type of rest that you might need between sets of weight-lifting exercises. It's much shorter and for a completely different reason. A person rests in between sets of weight-lifting exercises to allow certain chemical changes to occur within the muscle. This recovery period prepares you for the next set. The Function First exercises don't require that kind of recovery. The rest period between your exercises has more to do with your being able to recognize what a muscle feels like when it's turned "on" and when it's turned "off." For example, if an exercise requires 3 sets of 15 repetitions (3 x 15), and you're working at 50 to 60 percent of what your perceived maximum would be, you might not feel as if you're working that hard. So you decide that you'll do 45 continuous repetitions, instead of breaking it up into 3 sets. If you do this, you'll end up holding the muscle in a continuous state of tension, even though you may feel as if you have released it in between your efforts. You may have reduced tension relative to the effort required, but you won't be able to reproduce the state of relaxation that the muscle would have in an inactive state. It's extremely important for your body to be able to recognize this difference. You don't want muscle tension to be background noise. If a muscle is tense for any number of reasons, we want you to be able to recognize this, so that you can take steps to intervene. You don't want to ignore it until you become used to it, and it becomes another page in another chapter of that history book that makes up you.

The next section of the book contains exercises for your Form and Category. It will be helpful if you prepare your exercise environment before you begin. You don't want to have to run for a pillow or move a coffee table or do anything like that while you're in the middle of exercising. Remember, it's best that you be "present" while doing your program. This means being conscious of what your body does and feels. Let your mind observe and experience the exercises along with your body to heighten the sensory experience. This will make your exercises that much more beneficial. Being glued to every word Oprah says while you do these exercises is less beneficial. Also, please remember to do the exercises in the order that they appear.

People often ask, "When is the best time of the day to do the exercises?" Priority number one is that you find *any* time, as long as you do them every day. If you have a choice, early in the day is recommended. Doing the exercises in the morning will allow you to integrate into your daily activities the structural and the neurological changes that the exercises stimulate. It also provides a line of defense against the daily activities that probably contribute to the overload of negative stimuli your body regularly receives. The exception to this would be if the exercises allowed you to sleep better at night and to make better use of that rejuvenation and healing time for your body.

At the end of all the Form and Category programs is the Graduate Program. You may advance to this program once you feel that you've corrected your Form through the associated exercise program. The Graduate Program is a more advanced routine that requires greater overall strength and neuromuscular coordination. Don't move on to the Graduate Program if you're still experiencing significant symptoms.

General Comments about the Exercises before You Begin

It is recommended that almost everyone should precede his or her exercise program with the 90-90 Neutral Back position. This position can be very comfortable for symptoms that are directly or indirectly related to the spine. It is more productive and beneficial for your body than simply lying down on your back with your legs straight or bent. The 90-90 name comes from the angle that must be present at the knee joints and at the hip joints. Stated another way, the upper leg must be perpendicular to the floor and the lower leg must be parallel to the floor. This position allows the muscles of the hips, the lower back, the upper back, the neck, and the shoulders to relax. When the muscles relax, it allows you to begin the exercises with a more neutral body position. In other words, it removes (albeit temporarily) the biases your body brings to the exercise session. For instance, if you do your exercises first thing in the morning after sleeping in a contorted position for eight hours, you'll bring some of that contortion into your exercise program if you don't neutralize things first. Or, if you do your exercises in the evening after a hard day and then a stressful ride home in traffic, the 90-90 Neutral Back will help you let go of that added muscle tension before you begin your exercise program.

The formal description of the 90-90 Neutral Back is as follows:

90-90 NEUTRAL BACK

Lie on your back with your legs draped over a chair or an ottoman. The height of the chair should allow your knees and hips to be bent to 90 degrees. Allow your arms to lie out to your sides on the floor, with the palms facing the ceiling. The arms should be placed about shoulder level. Relax in this position and allow the back muscles to relax.

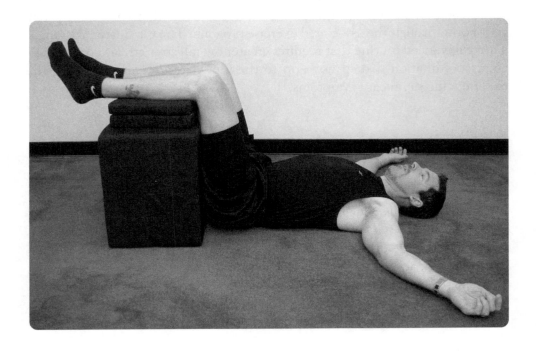

Recommended Duration

Approximately 3 to 10 minutes, or as needed to allow the body to relax.

Modification

Place a small rolled-up towel under your neck for comfort. If your head cannot lie flat on the floor, use a small pillow to support your head. *Note:* The long-term goal is to have your head on the floor without pain.

Purpose

To allow the muscles around the hips and the pelvis and along the spine to relax. This will let the body settle into a neutral, symmetrical position on the floor. The position is also very effective for the temporary relief of many aches and pains associated with the hips, the pelvis, and the spine.

The sets and the repetitions given with each exercise are recommendations. They can be increased or decreased slightly, based on your present physical conditioning. Remember, the purpose of this exercise program is not to exhaust the muscles but to remind them to do the job they were designed to do. So, if you feel overworked by a particular exercise, reduce the number of repetitions. Additional photos and views of the exercises can be found at www.movementbydesign.com.

Part Two
Regaining Control

8

Form 1 Exercises

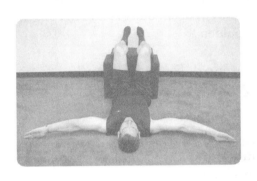

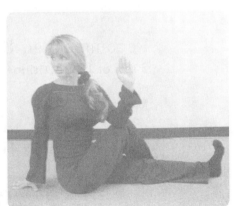

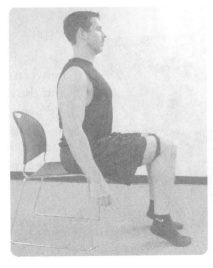

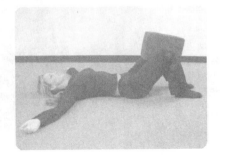

REVERSE BENCH PRESS IN 90-90 NEUTRAL BACK

Lie on your back, with your legs draped over a chair or an ottoman. Place your arms on the floor, at shoulder level. Bend the elbows to 90 degrees so that the wrists are directly over the elbows. Your hands are open, with the palms of the hands facing forward. From this position, gently press and release your elbows into the floor. This should cause your shoulder blades to come together. Do this without shrugging your shoulders.

Recommended Sets and Repetitions
3 sets of 15 repetitions

Modifications
If you feel this exercise in your neck, slightly lower your elbows toward your sides, to avoid using the neck muscles.

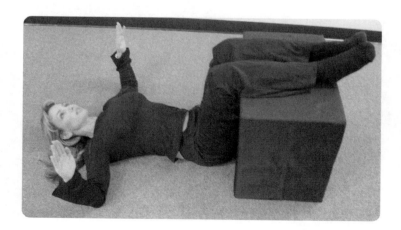

Purpose
To activate the muscles between the shoulder blades and the muscles of the middle/upper back. This assists in bringing the shoulders back to a more anatomically correct position.

ADDUCTOR SQUEEZES SUPINE

Lie on your back with your knees bent. Your feet should point straight ahead, and your feet, knees, and hips should be in a straight line. Your arms are out to the side on the floor with the palms facing up. Place a 6- to 8-inch ball or pillow between your knees. Gently, squeeze and release the pillow with your knees. You should feel this in your inner thighs.

Recommended Sets and Repetitions
3 sets of 20 repetitions

Modifications
None

Purpose
To activate the inner thigh muscles, which are important in pelvic stabilization. They also assist in the inward rotation of the thigh at the hip joint.

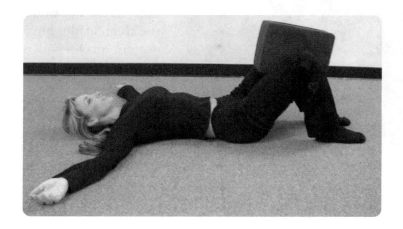

ABDUCTOR PRESSES SUPINE

Lie on your back with your knees bent. Your feet should point straight ahead, and your feet, knees, and hips should be in a straight line. Place a non-elastic belt or strap around your thighs, just above the knees. Gently press out and release against the strap as if you were trying to separate your knees. You should feel this in your outer thighs and buttocks.

Recommended Sets and Repetitions
3 sets of 20 repetitions

Modifications
Bring your knees closer together before placing the strap around your thighs to help you feel the exercise in the right muscles.

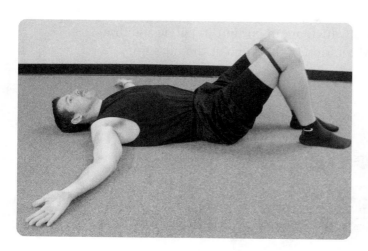

Purpose
To activate the outer thigh muscles, which are important in pelvic stabilization. They also assist in the outward rotation of the thigh at the hip joint. This exercise may assist in the positioning of your sacroiliac joint as well. The exercise should be felt in the outer thighs/hips and the buttocks.

HEEL LIFTS SITTING WITH STRAP

Sit on a firm chair that allows you to have your knees and hips bent to 90 degrees. Your feet should point straight ahead, and your feet, knees, and hips should be in a straight line. Place a non-elastic belt or strap around the thighs, just above the knees. Roll your pelvis forward, and sit tall on your "sit bones" under the buttocks. This should create an arch in your lower back. From this position, place a slight but constant pressure outward on the strap around your legs. While maintaining this sitting position and the pressure on the strap, lift and lower your heels off the floor. Do this by lifting from your top, upper-thigh muscles. Your calves will also be involved with this exercise, but we don't want them doing all of the work.

Recommended Sets and Repetitions
3 sets of 15 repetitions

Modifications
None

Purpose
To activate the hip flexor muscles, while keeping the proper alignment of your hips with the strap. The sitting posture also helps to assist in strengthening and building endurance in the stabilizers of the spine. This exercise should be felt predominantly on the tops of the thighs and the fronts of the hips.

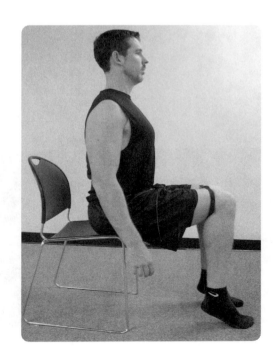

HIP ROTATOR STRETCH

Lie on your back with your feet flat on a wall and your knees and hips bent to a 90-degree angle. Cross the left ankle over the right knee. As you do this, it's extremely important that your hips stay square to the wall. The tendency is for the pelvis to rotate away if the hips are tight. Using the muscles of your left hip (not your hand), gently press the left knee away from your body toward the wall. Remember to keep your hips square on the floor. Hold this position for the desired amount of time. You should feel the stretch in the area of the left buttocks. Repeat with the opposite leg.

Recommended Duration
1 to 2 minutes

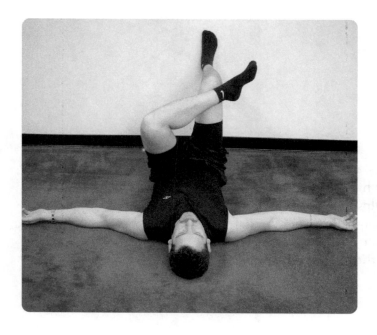

Modifications
If your hips are too tight and you cannot keep your hips square to the wall, place your feet on the floor instead of on the wall. Perform the stretch the same as described previously.

Purpose
To assist in positioning the hip joint by elongating the deep outward rotators of the hip. You should feel this stretch in the buttocks of the leg that has the crossed ankle.

SWAY-BACK POSE

Kneel on some books or cushions that are approximately 10 inches high. With your knees still on the lift, drop forward so that your hands are on the floor. Place your hands directly under your shoulders with the elbows straight. Viewed from the side, the hip joint should be just slightly in front of the knee joint. From this position, allow your stomach to relax and your back to sway. Also, allow your shoulder blades to collapse together while still keeping your elbows straight. Your head hangs down, and your neck should be relaxed. Your awareness should be in your upper and lower back.

Recommended Duration
1 to 2 minutes

Modifications
This exercise can be modified in three ways. The first would be to back your hips up over your knees to relieve some of the pressure from the lower back.

The second would be to do this exercise on the floor, without elevating the knees. The third would be to rest on your forearms with the elbows bent. Your elbows, instead of your hands, would then be directly under the shoulders.

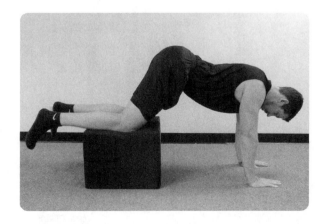

Purpose
To allow the spine to passively relax into a position of extension (the opposite of sitting slouched).

HEEL DROP ON STAIRS

Stand at the bottom of a stairwell or in a doorway with a platform comparable to the height of a single stair with the balls of your feet on the step. Your feet should be about 4 to 6 inches apart and pointing straight ahead. Place one hand on the nearest handrail, or stand in the middle and use both handrails if possible. Allow your heels to drop down. As you do this, it's very important that you keep your body aligned straight up and down, if viewed from the side. Imagine a straight line extending from your ear to your shoulder to your hip to your knee to your ankle. Don't bend forward at the waist, and don't allow your hips to move ahead of the rest of your body.

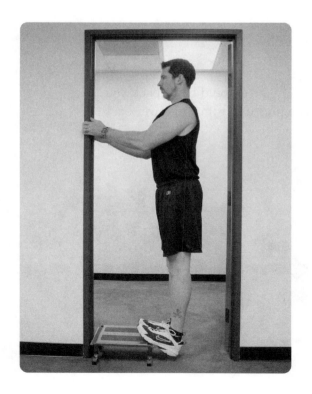

Recommended Duration
2 to 3 minutes

Modifications
To increase or decrease the amount of stretch in your calves, put more or less of your foot on the step.

Purpose
Although you'll feel an obvious stretch in your calves, this isn't the primary purpose of the exercise. By keeping the body aligned perfectly as described, you are using many of your postural muscles to maintain and "learn" this position.

STATIC SQUAT

Stand about an arm's length away from a pole, a banister, or two doorknobs. Grab hold at about waist level. Walk your feet in so that they are under your hands. Your feet should point straight ahead and be in line with your knees and hips. From this position, squat down to 90 degrees at your knees and hips. Keep your arms straight. Rotate your pelvis forward so that you are arching your lower back and flattening your upper back. Stick your chest out. Keep your eyes focused straight ahead and hold.

Recommended Duration
30 seconds to 1 minute

Modifications
Limit the depth of the squat slightly or decrease the time. Limiting the depth of the squat too much will decrease the value of the exercise considerably.

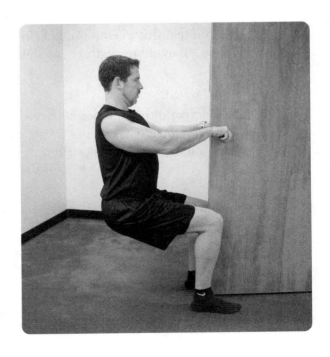

Purpose
To increase the static strength of the hip muscles and the spinal extensors. You should feel the thighs working, as well as the extensor muscles in your lower and upper back.

Program 1.2
Form 1, Category 2 (Dexterity Worker)

REVERSE BENCH PRESS IN 90-90 NEUTRAL BACK (see page 94)

Lie on your back, with your legs draped over a chair or an ottoman. Place your arms on the floor, at shoulder level. Bend your elbows to 90 degrees so that your wrists are directly over the elbows. Your hands are open, with the palms of the hands facing forward. From this position, gently press and release your elbows into the floor. This should cause your shoulder blades to come together. Do this without shrugging your shoulders.

Recommended Sets and Repetitions
3 sets of 15 repetitions

Modifications
If you feel this exercise in your neck, slightly lower your elbows toward your sides, to avoid using the neck muscles.

Purpose
To activate the muscles between the shoulder blades and the muscles of the middle/upper back. This assists in bringing the shoulders back to a more anatomically correct position.

SNOW ANGELS IN 90-90 NEUTRAL BACK

Lie on your back, with your legs draped over a chair or an ottoman. Rest your arms on the floor at your sides. Keep your fingers, wrists, and elbows straight. The little-finger-side of the hand will be the only part of the hand to touch the floor. Raise your arms along the floor, with your elbows straight up to shoulder level. At shoulder level, rotate your entire arm and hand back so that the thumb-side of the hand is touching the floor. From this position, bring your hands along the floor and overhead, keeping the elbows straight. Reverse the process on the way down. Lower your arms with the thumb-side on the floor until they're shoulder level. Rotate your arms forward so that the little-finger-side of the hand is on the floor, then return them along your sides and repeat.

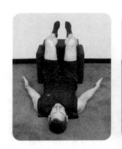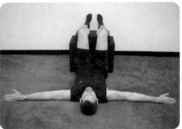

Recommended Sets and Repetitions
3 sets of 10 repetitions

Modifications
Limit how far overhead you go with your hands if you have to bend your elbows. Alternately, you may continue the overhead movement until your palms touch as long as your elbows remain straight.

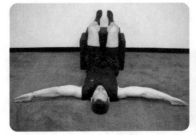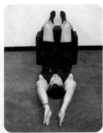

Purpose
First, to assist the body in recruiting the muscles that extend the upper back. In addition, to teach the body to coordinate the movement of the arm with the shoulder blade. You should feel the muscles of your shoulders and upper and middle back working. You may feel a stretch along your arms.

ANKLE ROCKING WITH STRAP

Lie on your back with your knees bent. Your feet should point straight ahead, and your feet, knees, and hips should be in a straight line. Place a non-elastic belt or strap around your thighs, just above the knees. Maintain a slight, constant pressure on the strap. Maintaining this position, lift the heels of both feet off the ground as high as you can. Keep the balls of your feet on the ground. Lower the heels back down, and raise the balls of your feet off the ground as high as you can while keeping the heels down. Rock back and forth, maintaining pressure on the strap.

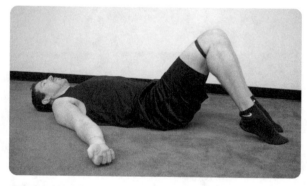

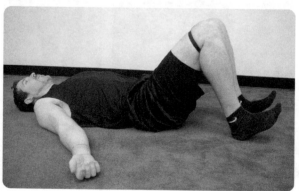

Recommended Sets and Repetitions
3 sets of 15 repetitions

Modifications
None

Purpose
To mimic the walking motion with your foot, while activating the stabilizers of your hip with the strap. You should feel this in the muscles of your lower leg and your hips.

UPPER SPINAL ROTATION

Lie on your side in the fetal position, with your hips and knees bent to 90 degrees. Your ankles, knees, hips, and shoulders should be stacked directly over one another. Place your bottom arm straight out on the floor at 90 degrees from your torso, and place the top hand on top of the bottom hand. From this position, rotate your top hand off your bottom hand toward the floor behind you. It's very important that you keep your knees together as you rotate. Let the weight of your top arm pull your body around. It's crucial to breathe, relax, and allow gravity to slowly bring your arm toward the floor. Your head should be relaxed on the floor, and your eyes should face the ceiling. After the desired time, slowly return to the starting position and repeat with the other side.

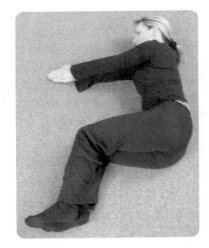

Recommended Duration
1 to 2 minutes

Modifications
If you have trouble keeping your knees together, reach down with your bottom hand to help hold your knees in place.

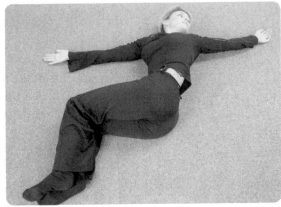

Purpose
To improve the spine's ability to rotate independently of the hips and the pelvis. You should feel a stretch across your chest and the top arm and a stretch along the side of your body and toward the lower back.

CAT AND DOG (see page 46)

Start on your hands and knees with your hands directly under your shoulders and your knees directly under your hips. Your body should be square, like a box. Your weight should be evenly distributed between all four points of contact. Relax your feet so that the tops of the feet rest on the floor. From this position, smoothly round up your back, draw your belly button toward your spine, and tuck your pelvis under. Drop your head and bring your chin toward your chest. From here, reverse directions by allowing your stomach to drop and your back to sway. Your shoulder blades should drop together and your head looks up. Make it one fluid movement, rather than holding any one position. Exhale as your head looks up, and inhale as your head looks down. It's important to keep your elbows straight as you perform the movement and to avoid rocking forward and backward at the hips and the shoulders.

Recommended Repetitions
15 repetitions

Modifications
You can limit the range of motion in either or both directions if you feel any restrictions or discomfort during the exercise.

Purpose
To improve motion of the entire spine, in both flexion and extension. It also provides a gentle stretch of the spinal flexors and extensors and helps with coordination of movement of the head and the pelvis.

ISOLATED HIP FLEXION SUPINE

Lie on your back with your knees bent. Your feet should point straight ahead and line up with your knees and hips. Your arms are out to the sides, with the palms facing the ceiling. From this position, lift one foot at a time 4 to 6 inches off the floor. Your foot should point straight ahead and remain directly in line with the knee and hip as you lift. Your back will want to rise (arch) off the floor as you lift. Use your abdominals to keep your lower back flat on the floor as you lift. Complete the recommended repetitions with one leg, and then repeat with the opposite leg. Alternate legs for each set.

Recommended Sets and Repetitions
3 sets of 15 repetitions

Modifications
If you experience discomfort in your lower back when raising the leg, place a rolled-up towel under your lower back for support.

Purpose
To reinforce proper tracking of the foot and the leg with the hip, as with walking. Also, to remind the abdominals of their role in stabilizing the pelvis while the hip flexor muscles are working. You should feel the work in your upper thigh toward the hip and in the abdominals.

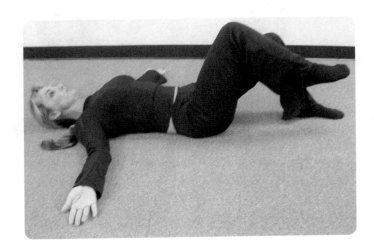

SIDE FOREARM STRETCH

Stand sideways to a wall. Place the palm of one hand against the wall at shoulder level. The fingers should point toward the ceiling. Stand far enough away so that your elbow is straight and your arm makes a 90-degree angle to the body. Your body should be perpendicular to the wall. Avoid shrugging the shoulder of the arm on the wall. Hold this position for the desired time. It's important that you keep the elbow straight and you maintain the proper alignment of your body. Switch sides and repeat.

Recommended Duration
45 seconds to 1 minute

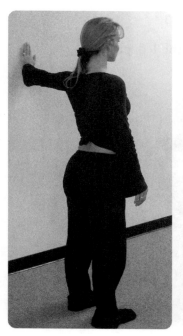 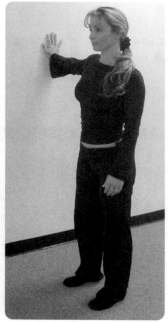

Modifications
None

Purpose
To elongate the muscles and the connective tissue that run the distance from the fingertips to the armpit. This will help to improve shoulder and hand posture. You should feel a stretch in the upper part of the forearm and maybe the hand.

SCAPULAR WALL PRESSES

Stand with your back to a wall. Your heels should be about 2 to 4 inches from the wall. Keep your buttocks, shoulders, and head against the wall. From this position, stretch your arms out straight against the wall, with the backs of your hands on the wall. Make your wingspan as long as possible. Your hands should be approximately halfway between your waist and shoulders. Press and release the backs of your hands into the wall. As you press, don't allow your buttocks, shoulders, or head to come off the wall. Avoid using your neck while pressing. Continue for the recommended number of repetitions.

Recommended Sets and Repetitions
3 sets of 10 repetitions

Modifications
If you feel the work in your neck or there is discomfort in your shoulders, lower your arms slightly toward the level of your waist.

Purpose
To combine strengthening of the spinal extensors and the muscles that bring the shoulder blades together. This is done by using the wall as a reference for alignment. You should feel this in the backs of the arms, in the upper back, and between the shoulder blades.

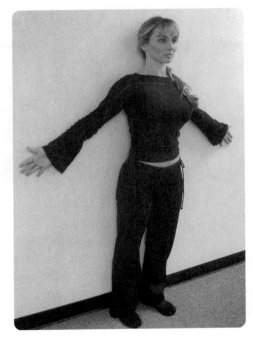

FOOT ROTATIONS IN 90-90 NEUTRAL BACK

Lie on your back with your arms extended on the floor at shoulder level, palms facing upward. Keep the lower leg still as it rests on a chair or an ottoman. Rotate one foot at a time in a clockwise direction. With your toes, draw as big a circle as you can in the air to maximize the range of motion at the ankle. After the desired repetitions, reverse directions by circling in a counterclockwise direction. After completing both directions, point your foot straight away from you and then pull your foot straight back toward you for the recommended repetitions. Repeat with the other foot. It's important to keep the lower leg still as you move the foot to ensure that the movement occurs at the ankle.

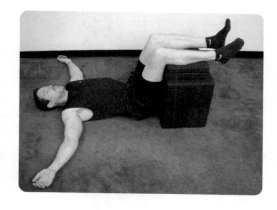

Recommended Sets and Repetitions

1 set of 20 repetitions for all three movements

Modifications

Decrease the number of repetitions if 20 is initially too challenging. Or, use alternate feet for each movement to rest one ankle as you work the other.

Purpose

The muscles at the foot and the ankle are critical for balance and will affect movements at the knees and the hips. This exercise takes those joints through all of their available ranges of motion and strengthens the muscles that are responsible. You should feel fatigue in the front and the sides of your shin muscles.

REVERSE BENCH PRESS IN 90-90 NEUTRAL BACK (see page 94)

Lie on your back, with your legs draped over a chair or an ottoman. Place your arms on the floor, at shoulder level. Bend your elbows to 90 degrees so that your wrists are directly over the elbows. Your hands are open, with the palms of the hands facing forward. From this position, gently press and release your elbows into the floor. This should cause your shoulder blades to come together. Do this without shrugging your shoulders.

Recommended Sets and Repetitions
3 sets of 15 repetitions

Modifications
If you feel this exercise in your neck, slightly lower your elbows toward your sides, to avoid using the neck muscles.

Purpose
To activate the muscles between the shoulder blades and the muscles of the middle/upper back. This assists in bringing the shoulders back to a more anatomically correct position.

SITTING SPINAL TWIST

Sit on the floor with your legs straight out in front of you. Sit as tall as you can. Cross your right foot over your left knee and place it flat on the floor alongside the left knee. Place your right hand on the floor behind you and close to your right buttocks for support. Pull the toes of your foot toward you and keep the left knee straight. Take your left elbow and place it across your body and against the outside of your right knee. As you remain sitting tall, rotate your head and shoulders to the right, attempting to look over your right shoulder. Hold this position for the desired length of time and breathe! Switch sides and repeat.

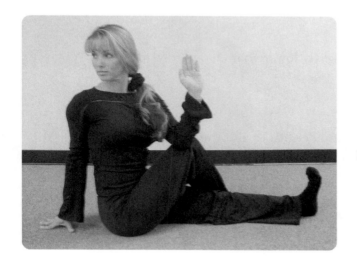

Recommended Duration
30 seconds to 1 minute

Modification
None

Purpose
To strengthen the spinal rotators, first on one side of the spine and then on the other side. You should feel a stretching along one side of your back and muscle contraction (shortening) along the other side of your back.

CAT AND DOG (see page 46)

Start on your hands and knees with your hands directly under your shoulders and your knees directly under your hips. Your body should be square, like a box. Your weight should be evenly distributed between all four points of contact. Relax your feet so that the tops of the feet rest on the floor. From this position, smoothly round up your back, draw your belly button toward your spine, and tuck your pelvis under. Drop your head and bring your chin toward your chest. From here, reverse directions by allowing your stomach to drop and your back to sway. Your shoulder blades should drop together and your head looks up. Make it one fluid movement, rather than holding any one position. Exhale as your head looks up and inhale as your head looks down. It's important to keep your elbows straight as you perform the movement and to avoid rocking forward and backward at the hips and shoulders. You should feel a movement of flexion and extension through your spine.

Recommended Repetitions
15 repetitions

Modifications
You can limit the range of motion in either or both directions if you feel any restrictions or discomfort during the exercise.

Purpose
To improve motion of the entire spine, in both flexion and extension. It also provides a gentle stretch of the spinal flexors and extensors and helps with coordinating movement of the head and the pelvis.

WALL HAMSTRING STRETCH

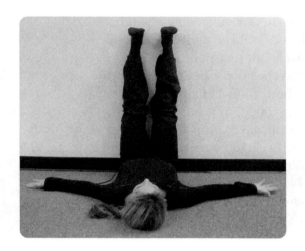

Lie on your back on the floor next to a wall. Place your legs straight up the wall with your feet, knees, and hips in line. Your body should be perpendicular to the wall. Ideally, your buttocks will be touching the wall. With your legs straight, pull the tops of your feet and toes back toward you. Tighten your front thigh muscles to straighten the knees. The upper buttocks area and the lower back should be resting firmly on the floor. Your arms are relaxed out to the sides, with the palms facing the ceiling. Hold this position for the recommended duration. You should feel a stretch in your calves and the backs of your thighs (hamstrings). Remember, a muscle stretch should not be so intense that it is painful. If this is the case, see the following modification.

Recommended Duration
1 to 1½ minutes

Modification
Move your buttocks away from the wall enough to be able to tolerate the stretch or to allow your upper buttocks and lower back to rest on the floor.

Purpose
To symmetrically lengthen the posterior muscles of the legs without the influence of the spinal muscles. Pulling the feet back and tightening the quadriceps helps to improve the efficiency of the stretch. You should feel the stretch in your calves and the backs of your thighs (hamstrings).

WALL HAMSTRING STRETCH WITH FEMUR ROTATIONS

Lie on your back on the floor next to a wall. Place your legs straight up the wall with your feet about 18 inches apart. Your body should be perpendicular to the wall. Ideally, your buttocks will be touching the wall. With your legs straight, pull the tops of your feet and toes back toward you. Tighten the front thigh muscles to straighten the knees. Your upper buttocks area and lower back should be resting firmly on the floor. Your arms are relaxed out to the sides, with the palms facing the ceiling. From this position, rotate both of your entire legs (not just your feet) toward each other. Then rotate them away from each other. Rotate only as far as you can while keeping the front thigh muscles tight. Think about the entire leg moving as if it were one unit. Continue rotating back and forth in a continuous smooth motion for the recommended repetitions.

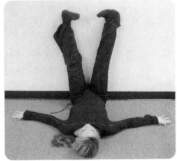

Recommended Sets and Repetitions
3 sets of 10 repetitions

Modifications
Move your buttocks away from the wall enough to be able to tolerate the stretch or to allow your upper buttocks and lower back to rest on the floor.

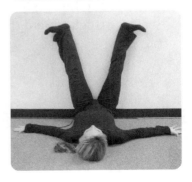

Purpose
To teach the body how to move the hip joints independently of the pelvis. It also strengthens the muscles that rotate the hip in and out. You should feel the movement occurring from around the hip joints. You may feel a slightly different stretch than you felt in the Wall Hamstring Stretch.

ISOLATED HIP FLEXION SUPINE (see page 107)

Lie on your back with your knees bent. Your feet should point straight ahead and line up with your knees and hips. Your arms are out to the sides with the palms facing the ceiling. From this position, lift one foot at a time 4 to 6 inches off the floor. Your foot should point straight ahead and remain directly in line with the knee and the hip as you lift. Your back will want to rise (arch) off the floor as you lift. Use your abdominals to keep your lower back flat on the floor as you lift. Complete the recommended repetitions with one leg, and then repeat with the opposite leg. Alternate legs for each set.

Recommended Sets and Repetitions
3 sets of 15 repetitions

Modifications
If you experience discomfort in your lower back when raising the leg, place a rolled-up towel under your lower back for support.

Purpose
To reinforce proper tracking of the foot and the leg with the hip, as with walking. Also, to remind the abdominals of their role in stabilizing the pelvis while the hip flexor muscles are working. You should feel the work in your upper thigh toward the hip and in the abdominals.

STATIC SQUAT (see page 101)

Stand about an arm's length away from a pole, a banister, or two doorknobs. Grab hold at about waist level. Walk your feet in so that they are under your hands. Your feet should point straight ahead and be in line with your knees and hips. From this position, squat down to 90 degrees at your knees and hips. Keep your arms straight. Rotate your pelvis forward so that you are arching your lower back and flattening your upper back. Stick your chest out. Keep your eyes focused straight ahead and hold.

Recommended Duration
30 seconds to 1 minute

Modifications
Limit the depth of the squat slightly or decrease the time. Limiting the depth of the squat too much will decrease the value of the exercise considerably.

Purpose
To increase the static strength of the hip muscles and the spinal extensors. You should feel the thighs working, as well as the extensor muscles in your lower and upper back.

9

Form 2 Exercises

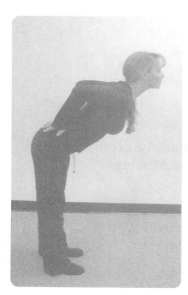

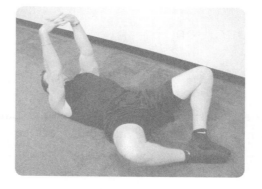

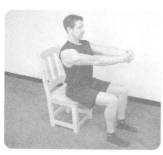

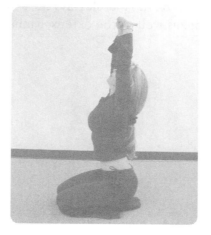

DOUBLE-ARM DOORWAY STRETCH

Stand in a doorjamb with one foot inside the doorjamb and one foot outside of it. Place the palms of your hands and your forearms on the doorjamb so that your elbows are bent to 90 degrees. The upper arms should be level with the shoulders. Tighten your abdominal muscles. Keep your chest high, and avoid shrugging your shoulders. Then lean your upper body through the doorjamb until you feel the stretch in your chest area. Hold this position for the recommended duration. After your first hold, relax, then switch the front and the back foot placement and repeat.

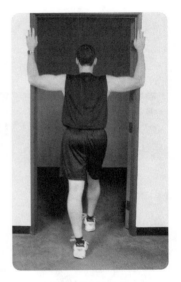

Recommended Sets and Duration

2 sets of 30 seconds

Modifications

Slightly vary the height of the elbow position to change the emphasis of the area stretched or to relieve any discomfort in the shoulders.

Purpose

To lengthen the muscles of the chest and the front shoulders, which will help to "open" the chest area. The stretch should be felt across your chest and front shoulders.

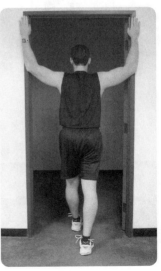

HIP ABDUCTION/ADDUCTION

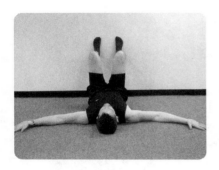

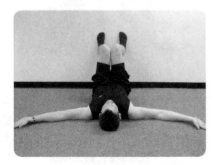

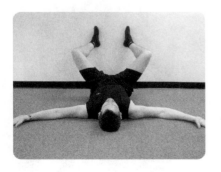

Lie on the floor with the bottoms of your feet on a wall. Lie so that your knees and hips are bent to a 90-degree angle. Your arms are out to the sides, with the palms facing the ceiling. From this position, bring your knees together so that they touch, and then spread them apart as far as you can. It is a smooth and controlled movement. The length of your foot must maintain contact with the wall during the movement. It's okay for you to roll to the outside edges of your feet. Keep your feet and toes pointing straight to the ceiling throughout the movement. Do not allow your heels to come off the wall.

Recommended Sets and Repetitions
2 sets of 20 repetitions

Modifications
Bringing your feet closer together will make it more challenging to get your knees apart. Placing your feet farther apart on the wall will make it more challenging to bring your knees together.

Purpose
To improve the ability of the hip to rotate in combination with movement of the thigh toward the body and away from the body. This movement is independent of the movement of the pelvis. You should feel this in your inner and outer thighs.

HIP ROTATOR STRETCH (see page 98)

Lie on your back with your feet flat on a wall and your knees and hips bent to a 90-degree angle. Cross the left ankle over the right knee. As you do this, it's extremely important that your hips stay square to the wall. The tendency is for the pelvis to rotate away if the hips are tight. Using the muscles of your left hip (not your hand), gently press the left knee away from your body toward the wall. Remember to keep your hips square on the floor. Hold this position for the desired amount of time. You should feel the stretch in the area of the left buttocks. Repeat with the opposite leg.

Recommended Duration
1 to 2 minutes

Modifications
If your hips are too tight and you cannot keep them square to the wall, place your feet on the floor instead of on the wall. Perform the stretch the same as described previously.

Purpose
To assist in positioning the hip joint by elongating the deep outward rotators of the hip. This stretch should be felt in the buttocks of the leg with the ankle crossed.

OPPOSITE ARM AND LEG GLIDING

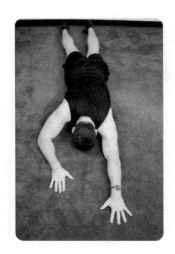

Lie facedown on the floor. Place a small folded towel or a washcloth under your forehead to keep your face off the floor. Lie with your arms straight out above your head and your legs in line with your hips. From this position, you will attempt to lengthen your body on opposite sides by reaching in a direct line with your body along the floor with one arm and in the opposite direction with the opposite leg. Hold this position for 5 seconds and relax. Repeat the movement with the other arm and leg. For each repetition, alternate the sides that you are reaching with. While you reach, it's very important that you remain in contact with the floor. Don't lift your arms or your hips as you reach. Imagine that you are moving on a sheet of ice. You should feel a stretch on the side of the lower back of the leg that is reaching, as well as muscular contraction around your upper back and the shoulder of the arm that is reaching.

Recommended Repetitions and Duration
Hold for 5 seconds for 10 repetitions on each side, alternating sides on each repetition.

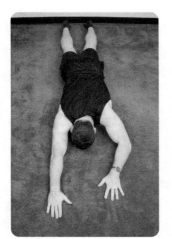

Modifications
If you experience discomfort in your shoulder, reach on a slight angle away from the body, instead of in a direct line with the body.

Purpose
To work the small, intrinsic muscles that stabilize the spine. This exercise also requires reciprocal movement of the upper and the lower body, similar to walking.

ADDUCTOR SQUEEZES SITTING

Sit on a firm chair that allows you to have your knees and hips bent to 90 degrees. Your feet should point straight ahead, and your feet, knees, and hips should be in a straight line. Roll your pelvis forward, and sit tall on your "sit bones" under the buttocks. This should create an arch in your lower back. Place a 6- to 8-inch ball or pillow between your knees. Allow your arms to hang relaxed at your sides. Gently squeeze and release the pillow with your knees. Do not lose the proper sitting position as you squeeze. You should feel muscles working in your inner thighs and lower back.

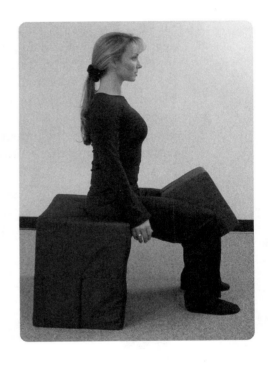

Recommended Sets and Repetitions
3 sets of 20 repetitions

Modifications
If the sitting position is too challenging or painful, attempt the exercise lying on your back with the knees bent.

Purpose
To activate the inner thigh muscles, which are important in pelvic stabilization. They also assist in the inward rotation of the thigh at the hip joint. This exercise strengthens the spinal stabilizers to maintain the sitting posture. The exercise should be felt in the inner thighs/hips and the lower back.

ABDUCTOR PRESSES SITTING

Sit on a firm chair that allows you to have your knees and hips bent to 90 degrees. Your feet should point straight ahead, and your feet, knees, and hips should be in a straight line. Roll your pelvis forward, and sit tall on your "sit bones" under the buttocks. This should create an arch in your lower back. Place a non-elastic belt or strap around your thighs, just above the knees. Gently press out and release against the strap, as if you were trying to separate your knees. Don't lose the proper sitting position as you press out. You should feel this in your outer thighs and buttocks.

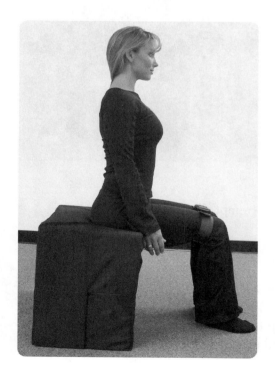

Recommended Sets and Repetitions
3 sets of 20 repetitions

Modifications
Bring your knees closer together before placing the strap around the thighs to help you feel the exercise in the right muscles. If the sitting position is too challenging or painful for you, attempt the exercise lying on your back with your knees bent.

Purpose
To activate the outer thigh muscles, which are important in pelvic stabilization. They also assist in the outward rotation of the thigh at the hip joint. This exercise strengthens the spinal stabilizers to maintain the sitting posture. The exercise should be felt in the outer thighs/hips, the buttocks, and the lower back.

SWAY-BACK ANKLE SQUEEZES

Kneel on the floor. Place an approximately 6-inch pillow or ball between your ankles. Drop forward so that you are on your hands and knees. If viewed from the side, your hip joints should be slightly ahead of the knee joints and your shoulders should be directly over the hands. Your fingers should point straight ahead. Relax the abdominal muscles and allow your back to drop into a sway-back position. Keep your elbows straight. Allow your head to hang down. Gently squeeze and release the pillow between your ankles, using the inner ankle bones and the inside borders of the feet. You should feel a contraction around your hips and buttocks. Continue for the desired number of sets and repetitions. When resting between sets, rest only from the squeezing; maintain the sway-back position while you rest from the squeezing.

Recommended Sets and Repetitions
3 sets of 20 repetitions

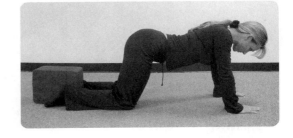

Modifications
This exercise can be modified in two ways. The first would be to back the hips up over the knees to relieve some of the pressure from the lower back. The second would be to rest on the forearms with the elbows bent. The elbows, instead of the hands, would then be directly under the shoulders.

Purpose
To strengthen the muscles of the hips while the lower back is in a position of passive extension. You should feel a contraction around your hips and the buttocks.

TABLE TOP WALL STRETCH

Stand facing a wall with your feet, knees, and hips all in alignment. Stand a little more than an arm's length away from the wall. Lean forward and reach out, placing the palms of your hands on the wall at approximately shoulder height. Straighten your elbows. Kick your buttocks backward, and allow your torso to drop down between your arms. You should bend from the hip joints and move your torso down between your arms as a unit. This should increase the arch in your back. Tighten your quadriceps (front thighs) and hold for the desired length of time.

Recommended Duration
1 minute

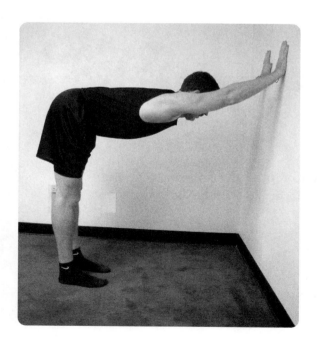

Modifications
Place your hands higher up on the wall and limit the distance you drop your torso down between your arms.

Purpose
To lengthen the muscles on the back side of the leg, while shortening the muscles of the back. Your arms on the wall assist in keeping your back in extension while the backs of the thighs lengthen. You should feel the stretch in your hamstrings (back of the thighs) and calves. You may also feel a stretch alongside your torso and a tightening in the upper back.

DOUBLE-ARM DOORWAY STRETCH (see page 119)

Stand in a doorjamb with one foot inside the doorjamb and one foot outside of it. Place the palms of your hands and your forearms on the doorjamb so that your elbows are bent to 90 degrees. The upper arms should be level with the shoulders. Tighten your abdominal muscles. Keep your chest high, and avoid shrugging your shoulders. Then lean your upper body through the doorjamb until you feel the stretch in your chest area. Hold this position for the recommended duration. After your first hold, relax, then switch the front and the back foot placement and repeat.

Recommended Sets and Duration

2 sets of 30 seconds

Modifications

Slightly vary the height of the elbow position to change the emphasis of the area stretched or to relieve any discomfort in the shoulders.

Purpose

To lengthen the muscles of the chest and the front shoulders, which will help to "open" the chest area. The stretch should be felt across your chest and front shoulders.

FROG PULLOVERS

Lie on your back on the floor. Bring the soles of your feet together, and as you do this, allow your knees to fall out to the sides. Pull your feet toward your groin, making sure that your feet are centered in the middle of your body. Allow gravity to pull your knees toward the floor. Don't try to push your knees down and don't resist if they drop. The lower back doesn't have to be flat on the floor, and you shouldn't feel pain in the back. Next, reach your arms straight out above your chest. Clasp your hands together and keep the elbows

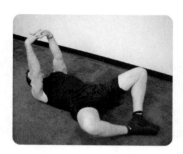

straight. From this position, bring your clasped hands overhead toward the floor behind you. Go only as far back as you can while keeping your elbows straight. If your elbows bend, stop at that point and return to the start. Repeat the overhead movement, using a slow, controlled motion. Repeat for the recommended sets and repetitions.

Recommended Sets and Repetitions
3 sets of 10 repetitions

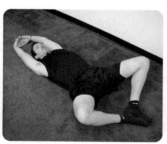

Modifications
If there is any discomfort or any limitation in the shoulder joints, keep the movement of the arms in a pain-free range.

Purpose
To increase the extension in the lower- and the upper-back areas and improve the position of the shoulder joints in relation to the upper back. You should feel a stretch in the inner thigh muscles and an increase in the arch throughout your back as your hands draw closer to the floor. You may also feel some muscular effort around the shoulder joints.

SCAPULAR WALL PRESSES (see page 109)

Stand with your back to a wall. Your heels should be about 2 to 4 inches from the wall. Keep your buttocks, shoulders, and head against the wall. From this position, stretch your arms out straight against the wall, with the backs of your hands on the wall. Make your wingspan as long as possible. Your hands should be approximately halfway between your waist and shoulders. Press and release the backs of your hands into the wall. As you press, don't allow your buttocks, shoulders, or head to come off the wall. Avoid using your neck while pressing. Continue for the recommended number of repetitions.

Recommended Sets and Repetitions
3 sets of 10 repetitions

Modifications
If you feel the work in your neck or there is discomfort in your shoulders, lower your arms slightly toward the level of your waist.

Purpose
To combine strengthening of the spinal extensors and the muscles that bring the shoulder blades together. This is done by using the wall as a reference point for alignment. You should feel this in the backs of the arms, in the upper back, and between the shoulder blades.

FORM 2 EXERCISES   129

SWAY-BACK ANKLE SQUEEZES (see page 125)

Kneel on the floor. Place an approximately 6-inch pillow or ball between your ankles. Drop forward so that you are on your hands and knees. If viewed from the side, your hip joints should be slightly ahead of the knee joints and your shoulders should be directly over the hands. Your fingers should point straight ahead. Relax the abdominal muscles and allow your back to drop into a sway-back position. Keep your elbows straight. Allow your head to hang down. Gently squeeze and release the pillow between your ankles, using the inner ankle bones and the inside borders of the feet. You should feel a contraction around your hips and buttocks. Continue for the desired number of sets and repetitions. When resting between sets, rest only from the squeezing. Maintain the sway-back position while you rest from the squeezing.

Recommended Sets and Repetitions
3 sets of 20 repetitions

Modifications
This exercise can be modified in two ways. The first would be to back the hips up over the knees to relieve some of the pressure from the lower back. The second would be to rest on the forearms with the elbows bent. The elbows, instead of the hands, would then be directly under the shoulders.

Purpose
To strengthen the muscles of the hips while the lower back is in a position of passive extension. You should feel a contraction around your hips and buttocks.

HERO'S POSE WITH OVERHEAD EXTENSION

Kneel on the floor with your feet and knees together. The tops of the feet should be flat on the floor. Sit back on your heels. Keep your shoulders over your hips, and avoid leaning forward. Next, tilt your pelvis forward, creating an arch in your lower back. Your shoulders should still be over your hips and not leaning forward. From this position, interlock your fingers together and raise your arms overhead, pushing the palms of your hands toward the ceiling. Look up at your hands and hold this position for the recommended time. You should feel this in your upper and middle back areas. You may also feel a stretch under the arms and on the tops of the thighs.

Recommended Duration

45 seconds to 1 minute

Modifications

If you lack flexibility in your feet, a rolled-up towel can be placed under the front part of your ankles, to minimize how much your feet have to flatten out. If you feel pressure in your knees, or there is too much stretch in the front of your thighs, place a thin couch pillow behind your knees.

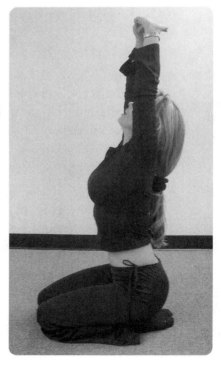

Purpose

To improve the strength and the endurance of the spinal extensor muscles and to teach the body awareness of the relationship between the pelvis and the spine.

ABDUCTOR PRESSES SITTING (see page 124)

Sit on a firm chair that allows you have your knees and hips bent to 90 degrees. Your feet should point straight ahead, and your feet, knees, and hips should be in a straight line. Roll your pelvis forward, and sit tall on your "sit bones" under the buttocks. This should create an arch in your lower back. Place a non-elastic belt or strap around your thighs, just above the knees. Gently press out and release against the strap, as if you were trying to separate your knees. Don't lose the proper sitting position as you press out. You should feel this in your outer thighs and buttocks.

Recommended Sets and Repetitions
3 sets of 20 repetitions

Modifications
Bring your knees closer together before placing the strap around your thighs to help you feel the exercise in the right muscles. If the sitting position is too challenging or painful for you, attempt the exercise lying on your back with your knees bent.

Purpose
To activate the outer thigh muscles, which are important in pelvic stabilization. They assist in the outward rotation of the thigh at the hip joint. This exercise strengthens the spinal stabilizers to maintain the sitting posture. The exercise should be felt in the outer thighs/hips, the buttocks, and the lower back.

PULLOVERS SITTING

Sit on a firm chair that allows you to have your knees and hips bent to 90 degrees. Your feet should point straight ahead, and your feet, knees, and hips should be in a straight line. Roll your pelvis forward, and sit tall on your "sit bones" under the buttocks. This should create an arch in your lower back. Hold your arms straight out from the shoulders and parallel to the floor. Clasp your fingers together. From this position, raise your arms overhead, keeping the elbows straight. Go overhead only as far as you can while keeping the elbows straight. Follow your hands with your eyes. Without pausing, return to the starting position, and repeat for the recommended sets and repetitions. You should feel the muscles of the upper and the lower back working during this exercise.

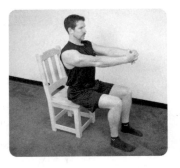

Recommended Sets and Repetitions
3 sets of 15 repetitions

Modifications
If there is any discomfort or limitation in your shoulder joints, keep the movement of the arms in a pain-free range. If you feel discomfort in your neck with the head movement, continue the exercise while keeping your eyes focused straight ahead.

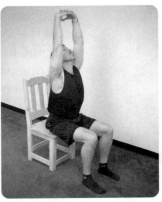

Purpose
To activate the spinal muscles, which improve shoulder position. Movement of the arms in this position improves the relationship of the shoulders and the upper back and helps to restore proper positioning of the shoulders. You should feel the muscles of your upper and lower back and shoulders working during this exercise.

TABLE TOP WALL STRETCH (see page 126)

Stand facing a wall with your feet, knees, and hips all in alignment. Stand a little more than an arm's length away from the wall. Lean forward and reach out placing the palms of your hands on the wall at approximately shoulder height. Straighten your elbows. Kick your buttocks backward and allow your torso to drop down between your arms. You should bend from the hip joints and move your torso down between your arms as a unit. This should increase the arch in your back. Tighten your quadriceps (front thighs) and hold for the desired length of time.

Recommended Duration
1 minute

Modifications
Place your hands higher up on the wall and limit the distance you drop your torso down between your arms.

Purpose
To lengthen the muscles on the back side of the leg, while shortening the muscles of the back. Your arms on the wall assist in keeping your back in extension while the backs of the thighs lengthen. You should feel the stretch in your hamstrings (back of the thighs) and calves. You may also feel a stretch alongside your torso and a tightening in the upper back.

DOUBLE-ARM DOORWAY STRETCH (see page 119)

Stand in a doorjamb with one foot inside the doorjamb and one foot outside of it. Place the palms of your hands and your forearms on the doorjamb so that your elbows are bent to 90 degrees. The upper arms should be level with the shoulders. Tighten your abdominal muscles. Keep your chest high, and avoid shrugging your shoulders. Then lean your upper body through the doorjamb until you feel the stretch in your chest area. Hold this position for the recommended duration. After your first hold, relax, then switch the front and the back foot placement and repeat.

Recommended Sets and Duration
2 sets of 30 seconds

Modifications
Slightly vary the height of the elbow position to change the emphasis of the area stretched or to relieve any discomfort in the shoulders.

Purpose
To lengthen the muscles of the chest and the front shoulders, which will help to "open" the chest area. The stretch should be felt across your chest and front shoulders.

HIP ABDUCTION/ADDUCTION (see page 120)

Lie on the floor with the bottoms of your feet on a wall. Lie so that your knees and hips are bent to a 90-degree angle. Your arms are out to the sides, with the palms facing the ceiling. From this position, bring your knees together so that they touch, and then spread them apart as far as you can. It is a smooth and controlled movement. The length of your foot must maintain contact with the wall during the movement. It's okay for you to roll to the outside edges of your feet. Keep your feet and toes pointing straight to the ceiling throughout the movement. Don't allow your heels to come off the wall.

Recommended Sets and Repetitions
2 sets of 20 repetitions

Modifications
Bringing your feet closer together will make it more challenging to get your knees apart. Placing your feet farther apart on the wall will make it more challenging to bring your knees together.

Purpose
To improve the ability of the hip to rotate in combination with movement of the thigh toward the body and away from the body. This movement is independent of movement of the pelvis. You should feel this in your inner and outer thighs.

HIP ROTATOR STRETCH (see page 98)

Lie on your back with your feet flat on a wall and your knees and hips bent to a 90-degree angle. Cross the left ankle over the right knee. As you do this, it's extremely important that your hips stay square to the wall. The tendency is for the pelvis to rotate away if the hips are tight. Using the muscles of your right hip (not your hand), gently press the right knee away from your body toward the wall. Remember to keep your hips square on the floor. Hold this position for the desired amount of time. You should feel the stretch in the area of the right buttocks. Repeat with the opposite leg.

Recommended Duration
1 to 2 minutes

Modifications
If your hips are too tight and you cannot keep your hips square to the wall, place your feet on the floor instead of on the wall. Perform the stretch the same as described previously.

Purpose
To assist in positioning the hip joint by elongating the deep outward rotators of the hip. This stretch should be felt in the buttocks of the leg with the ankle crossed.

OPPOSITE ARM AND LEG GLIDING (see page 122)

Lie facedown on the floor. Place a small folded towel or a washcloth under your forehead to keep your face off the floor. Lie with your arms straight out above your head and your legs in line with your hips. From this position, you will attempt to lengthen your body on opposite sides by reaching in a direct line with your body along the floor with one arm and in the opposite direction with the opposite leg. Hold this position for 5 seconds and relax. Repeat the movement with the other arm and leg. For each repetition, alternate the sides that you are reaching with. While you reach, it's very important that you remain in contact with the floor. Don't lift your arms or your hips as you reach. Imagine that you are moving on a sheet of ice. You should feel a stretch on the side of the lower back of the leg that is reaching, as well as muscular contraction around your upper back and the shoulder of the arm that is reaching.

Recommended Repetitions and Duration
Hold for 5 seconds for 10 repetitions on each side, alternating sides on each repetition.

Modifications
If you experience discomfort in your shoulder, reach on a slight angle away from the body instead of in a direct line with the body.

Purpose
To work the small, intrinsic muscles that stabilize the spine. This exercise also requires reciprocal movement of the upper and the lower body, similar to walking.

ISOLATED HIP FLEXION SUPINE (see page 107)

Lie on your back with your knees bent. Your feet should point straight ahead and line up with your knees and hips. Your arms are out to the sides, with the palms facing the ceiling. From this position, lift one foot at a time 4 to 6 inches off the floor. Your foot should point straight ahead and remain directly in line with the knee and the hip as you lift. Your back will want to rise (arch) off the floor as you lift. Use your abdominals to keep your lower back flat on the floor as you lift. Complete the recommended repetitions with one leg, and then repeat with the opposite leg. Alternate legs for each set.

Recommended Sets and Repetitions
3 sets of 15 repetitions

Modifications
If you experience discomfort in your lower back when raising the leg, place a rolled-up towel under your lower back for support.

Purpose
To reinforce proper tracking of the foot and the leg with the hip, as with walking. Also, to remind the abdominals of their role in stabilizing the pelvis while the hip flexor muscles are working. You should feel the work in your upper thigh toward the hip and in the abdominals.

SWAY-BACK ANKLE SQUEEZES (see page 125)

Kneel on the floor. Place an approximately 6-inch pillow or ball between your ankles. Drop forward so that you are on your hands and knees. If viewed from the side, your hip joints should be slightly ahead of the knee joints and your shoulders should be directly over the hands. Your fingers should point straight ahead. Relax the abdominal muscles and allow your back to drop into a sway-back position. Keep your elbows straight. Allow your head to hang down. Gently squeeze and release the pillow between your ankles, using the inner ankle bones and the inside borders of the feet. You should feel a contraction around your hips and buttocks. Continue for the desired number of sets and repetitions. When resting between sets, rest only from the squeezing. Maintain the sway-back position while you rest from the squeezing.

Recommended Sets and Repetitions
3 sets of 20 repetitions

Modifications
This exercise can be modified in two ways. The first would be to back the hips up over the knees to relieve some of the pressure from the lower back. The second would be to rest on the forearms with the elbows bent. The elbows, instead of the hands, would then be directly under the shoulders.

Purpose
To strengthen the muscles of the hips while the lower back is in a position of passive extension.

140   THE PAIN-FREE PROGRAM

STANDING HIP HINGE

Stand with your feet hip-width apart and pointing straight ahead. Place your hands on your hips so that the thumbs are to the front over the hip bones and pointing down. The rest of your fingers should be resting on the upper buttocks and pointing toward the floor. Try to squeeze your elbows together and hold. Tighten your front thigh muscles. Keeping an arch in your lower back, bend forward and hinge from the hip joints. Bend only as far forward as you can without losing the arch in your lower back. Shift the weight toward the balls of your feet, and focus your eyes straight ahead. Hold for the recommended duration. You should feel a stretch in your calves and hamstrings. You may also feel the muscular effort in your lower back.

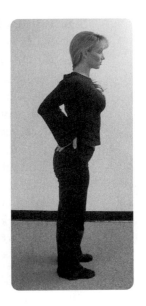

Recommended Duration
45 seconds to 1 minute

Modifications
Instead of placing your hands on your lower back, stand in front of a dining table or a desk and place your hands on that. Use your upper body to control how far you bend forward. It is still critical that you maintain the arch in your lower back and hinge from the hip as you lean forward.

Purpose
To lengthen the hamstring and calf muscles against gravity, while stabilizing the lumbar spine with the spinal extensor muscles.

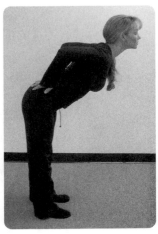

CAT AND DOG (see page 46)

Start on your hands and knees with your hands directly under your shoulders and your knees directly under your hips. Your body should be square, like a box. Your weight should be evenly distributed between all four points of contact. Relax your feet so that the tops of the feet rest on the floor. From this position, smoothly round up your back, draw your belly button toward your spine, and tuck your pelvis under. Drop your head and bring your chin toward your chest. From here, reverse directions by allowing your stomach to drop and your back to sway. Your shoulder blades should drop together and your head looks up. Make it one fluid movement, rather than holding any one position. Exhale as your head looks up, and inhale as your head looks down. It's important to keep your elbows straight as you perform the movement and to avoid rocking forward and backward at the hips and the shoulders. You should feel a movement of flexion and extension through your spine.

Recommended Repetitions
15 repetitions

Modifications
You can limit the range of motion in either or both directions if you feel any restrictions or discomfort during the exercise.

Purpose
To improve motion of the entire spine in both flexion and extension. It also provides a gentle stretch of the spinal flexors and extensors and helps with coordinating movement of the head and the pelvis.

10

Form 3 Exercises

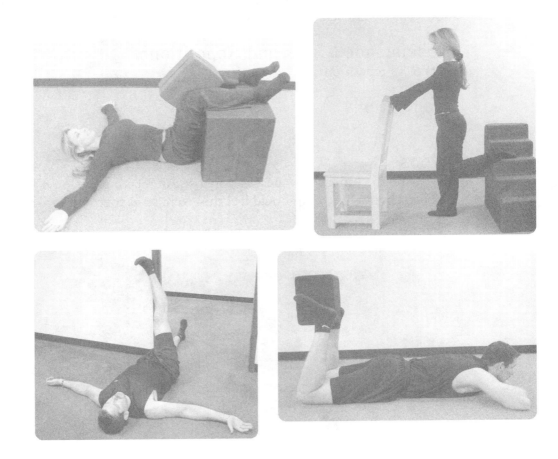

ADDUCTOR SQUEEZES IN THE 90-90 NEUTRAL BACK

Lie on your back, with your legs draped over a chair or an ottoman. Place a 6-inch ball or a firm pillow between your knees. Your knees should be elevated and in line with your hips. Relax your arms out to the sides, with the palms facing the ceiling. Gently squeeze and release the pillow with your knees. Don't allow your lower back to arch off the floor as you squeeze.

Recommended Sets and Repetitions
3 sets of 15 repetitions

Modifications
None

Purpose
To activate the inner thigh muscles and assist in relaxing the lower back and the buttocks muscles. You should feel this exercise in your inner thighs.

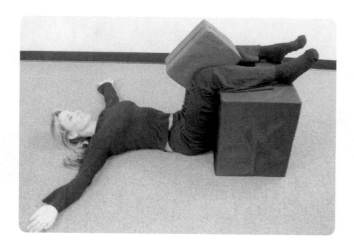

TVA DRAW ON ALL FOURS

Start on your hands and knees with your hands directly under your shoulders and your knees directly under your hips. Your body should be square, like a box. Your weight should be evenly distributed between all four points of contact. Relax your feet so that the tops of the feet rest on the floor. Allow gravity to pull your belly slightly toward the floor. We are trying to achieve a "neutral" spine, which means just a slight arch in the lower back. From this position, draw your belly button to your spine as if you were hollowing out your abdominal area. To use the appropriate muscles for this, you cannot move your spine or hips as you draw in. They should remain still. Once you have drawn all the way in, hold the contraction. You should feel the work toward the lower, inner part of the abdominals. You may even feel it in the deep pelvic floor muscles.

Recommended Duration and Repetitions
Hold for 3 seconds for 10 repetitions. Increase the hold time as you get more comfortable with the exercise.

Modifications
Lie on your back with your knees bent if you are unable to recruit the proper muscles in this exercise or are unable to perform the exercise without moving your hips and spine. Instead, draw your belly button to the floor, again without moving your hips.

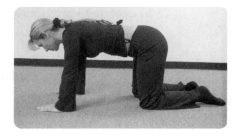

Purpose
To assist the body in using the deepest abdominal and "core" muscles for spinal stabilization. These muscles are underused in many people, who instead substitute with the more superficial abdominals.

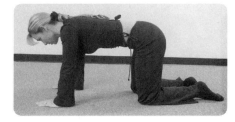

HIP ROTATOR STRETCH (see page 98)

Lie on your back with your feet flat on a wall and the knees and hips bent to a 90-degree angle. Cross the left ankle over the right knee. As you do this, it's extremely important that your hips stay square to the wall. The tendency is for the pelvis to rotate away if the hips are tight. Using the muscles of your left hip (not your hand), gently press the left knee away from the body toward the wall. Remember to keep the hips square on the floor. Hold this position for your desired amount of time. You should feel the stretch in the area of your right buttocks. Repeat with the opposite leg.

Recommended Duration
1 to 2 minutes

Modifications
If your hips are too tight and you cannot keep your hips square to the wall, place your feet on the floor instead of on the wall. Perform the stretch the same as described previously.

Purpose
To assist in positioning the hip joint by elongating the deep outward rotators of the hip. This stretch should be felt in the buttocks of the leg with the ankle crossed.

ANKLE SQUEEZES PRONE

Lie on your stomach with your hands on the floor and your chin resting on your hands. Grab hold of a 6- to 8-inch ball or pillow with your ankles. Bend your knees to 90 degrees, holding onto the ball. The 90-degree angle at the knees is a very important part of this exercise. From this position, gently squeeze and release the ball with your inner ankle bones and the inside borders of your feet. Don't squeeze with only the heels.

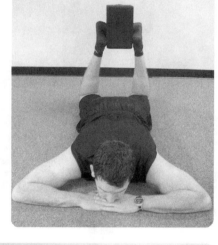

Recommended Sets and Repetitions
3 sets of 20 repetitions

Modifications
If you don't feel the contraction in your buttocks, spread your knees apart slightly until you do feel the work in the buttocks area. If you feel pressure or pain in your lower back with your knees bent, perform the exercise with your legs straight on the floor.

Purpose
To activate the buttocks muscles and the deep muscles under the buttocks. This improves the relationship of these muscles to the lower back and helps with hip alignment. The contraction should be felt in your buttocks area.

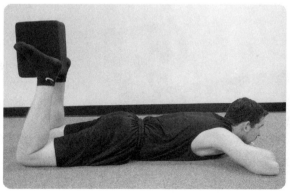

ISOLATED HAMSTRING STRETCH WITH CROSSOVER

Lie in a doorway with your outside thigh against the doorjamb and your legs straight. Lift your inside leg straight up and cross it over your body, placing the

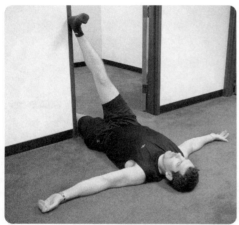

heel on the doorjamb. Keep the kneecap of the inside leg pointing straight off the doorjamb. Pull the foot and the toes of the leg on the doorjamb back toward you, and tighten the front thigh muscles. Your arms are out to the side, at chest level, with the palms facing the ceiling.

Recommended Duration
45 seconds to 1 minute

Modifications
You can move your body closer to the doorjamb or farther away from the doorjamb depending on your flexibility. Moving closer to the doorjamb will increase the stretch, and moving away from the doorjamb will decrease the stretch.

Purpose
To lengthen the hamstrings and the outer hip muscles independently of the lower back. You should feel the stretch of this exercise in your calf, hamstring, and buttock of the leg that's up and across the doorjamb.

LEG EXTENSIONS SUPINE

Lie on your back with your knees bent. Your feet, knees, and hips are in line, and your feet are pointing straight ahead. Your arms are out to the sides, with the palms facing the ceiling. Draw your belly button down to the floor and tighten all of your abdominal muscles to flatten your lower back entirely to the floor. While holding this position, lift one foot off the floor so that the lower leg from the knee down is parallel to the floor. The hip and the knee should be bent. Slowly straighten out this leg as you keep the lower leg parallel to the floor. Straighten the leg only as far as you can while keeping your lower back flat to the floor. When you feel your lower back arch off the floor, bring the leg back to the start and repeat. After the recommended repetitions for the first set, switch legs and repeat with the other leg.

Recommended Sets and Repetitions
3 sets of 5 repetitions

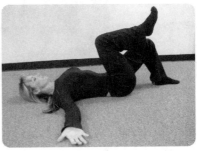

Modifications
If you are not able to keep your lower back flat on the floor at all as you begin to straighten your leg, then keep your feet on the floor. Maintain the required engagement of the abdominal muscles. Instead of lifting one foot, slide the heel away from your body, allowing your hip and knee to extend. Only slide the heel as far as you can while maintaining your flat back on the floor. Return to the start and repeat.

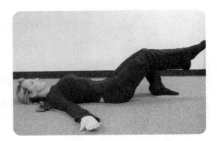

Purpose
To improve control of the abdominals and help them contribute to stabilizing the lower back and the pelvis. You should predominantly feel this exercise in the abdominal area.

KNEELING HIP FLEXOR STRETCH

Begin with one knee on the floor. Keep both legs in line with the hips. The foot of the front leg should be slightly in front of the knee of the same leg. The foot of the back leg should be directly in line with the knee of the back leg. Place

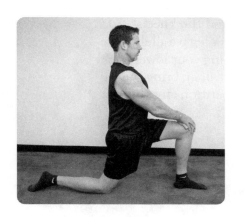

your hands on top of the thigh of the front leg, and keep your torso straight up and down. Tighten your abdominals and slightly tilt your pelvis backward, decreasing the arch in your lower back. Once you have done this, lunge slightly forward, bringing the front knee over the front ankle. Once in this position, lift the arm on the kneeling side of the body up and over the head for a side stretch. Keep your abdominals tight the entire time. Hold for the recommended duration, then repeat on the other side.

Recommended Duration
1 minute

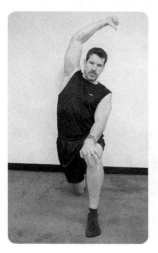

Modifications
If you are challenged with balance during this exercise, kneel next to a chair and place one hand on the chair to help you maintain your balance. Getting a proper stretch with this exercise is more important than the balance component. If your knee is uncomfortable, place a thin, flat pillow under it during the exercise.

Purpose
To lengthen the hip flexor muscles, which have a significant influence on the lower back. You should feel a stretch in the thigh and the groin of the back leg.

ANKLE SQUEEZES KNEELING

Kneel upright on the floor with your knees directly under your hips. The tops of your feet are flat on the floor. Place a 6- to 8-inch ball or pillow between your ankles. Allow your arms to hang at your sides. Gently squeeze and release the ball with your inner ankle bones and the inside borders of your feet. Don't squeeze with only the heels. The contraction should be felt in your buttocks area.

Recommended Sets and Repetitions
3 sets of 20 repetitions

Modifications
If you don't feel the contraction in the buttocks, spread your knees apart slightly until you do feel the work in the buttocks area. If you are challenged by holding yourself in this position, kneel in front of a chair and support yourself with the seat of the chair. Try to progress from using the chair for balance to balancing on your own.

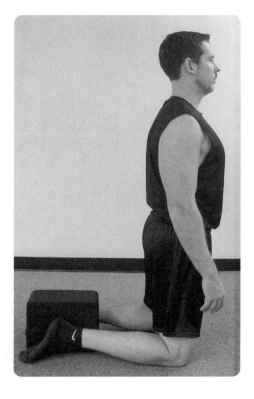

Purpose
To activate the gluteal muscles and help them to keep the pelvis in a neutral and upright balance.

Program 3.2
Form 3, Category 2 (Dexterity Work)

ADDUCTOR SQUEEZES IN THE 90-90 NEUTRAL BACK (see page 144)

Lie on your back, with your legs draped over a chair or an ottoman. Place a 6-inch ball or a firm pillow between your knees. Your knees should be in line with your hips. Relax your arms out to the sides with the palms facing the ceiling. Gently, squeeze and release the pillow with your knees. Don't allow your lower back to arch off the floor as you squeeze.

Recommended Sets and Repetitions
3 sets of 15 repetitions

Modifications
None

Purpose
To activate the inner thigh muscles and assist in relaxing the lower back and the buttocks muscles. You should feel this exercise in your inner thighs.

TVA DRAW ON ALL FOURS (see page 145)

Start on your hands and knees with your hands directly under your shoulders and your knees directly under your hips. Your body should be square, like a box. Your weight should be evenly distributed between all four points of contact. Relax your feet so that the tops of the feet rest on the floor. Allow gravity to pull your belly slightly toward the floor. We are trying to achieve a "neutral" spine, which means just a slight arch in the lower back. From this position, draw your belly button to your spine as if you were hollowing out your abdominal area. To use the appropriate muscles for this, you cannot move your spine or hips as you draw in. They should remain still. Once you have drawn all the way in, hold the contraction. You should feel the work toward the lower, inner part of the abdominals. You may even feel it in the deep pelvic floor muscles.

Recommended Duration and Repetitions

Hold for 3 seconds for 10 repetitions. Increase the hold time as you get more comfortable with the exercise.

Modifications

Lie on your back with your knees bent if you are unable to recruit the proper muscles in this exercise or are unable to perform the exercise without moving your hips and spine. Instead, draw your belly button to the floor, again without moving your hips.

Purpose

To assist the body in using the deepest abdominal and "core" muscles for spinal stabilization. These muscles are underused in many people, who instead substitute with the more superficial abdominals.

QUADRICEPS STRETCH STANDING

Stand facing the back of a chair at an arm's length away. Place a chair or an object with a comparable height and surface behind you. Stand with your feet pointing straight ahead and directly under your hips. Place the top of one foot on the back or the arm of the chair. The height of your foot placement determines how much stretch you feel in your front thigh muscles. When you first put your foot up on the chair, you should be aware of a mild stretch. Once you've got your foot on the chair, you must adjust your alignment. Make sure that both knees are aligned side to side. One should not be in front of the other. Place your hands on the chair in front of you to keep your torso straight up and down. From this position, you will rotate your pelvis posteriorly (tip the punch bowl backward). When you rotate your pelvis, you should feel an increase in the stretch in your front thigh muscles. Be careful not to push the pelvis forward instead of rotating the pelvis backward.

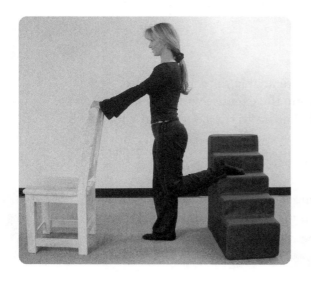

Recommended Duration
1 minute

Modifications
The height that the foot is propped up behind you dictates the stretch. Increase the height of your foot with a pillow to increase the stretch.

Purpose
To lengthen the quadriceps muscles and position the pelvis in neutral. This stretch should be felt from the knee to the front of the hip.

SIDE FOREARM STRETCH (see page 108)

Stand sideways to a wall. Place the palm of one hand against the wall at shoulder level. The fingers should point toward the ceiling. Stand far enough away so that your elbow is straight and your arm makes a 90-degree angle to the body. Your body should be perpendicular to the wall. Avoid shrugging the shoulder of the arm on the wall. Hold this position for the desired amount of time. It's important that you keep the elbow straight and you maintain the proper alignment of your body. Switch sides and repeat.

Recommended Duration
45 seconds to 1 minute

Modifications
None

Purpose
To elongate the muscles and the connective tissue that run the distance from the fingertips to the armpit. This will help to improve shoulder and hand posture. You should feel a stretch in the upper part of the forearm and maybe the hand.

ONE-ARM TABLE TOP STRETCH KNEELING

Kneel in front of a chair or a couch. Bend forward and place one hand on the floor under your shoulder and the other forearm on the chair. The elbow of the arm on the chair should be straight, with the thumb pointing to the ceiling. Tighten your abdominals so that your lower back is not arching toward the floor. Bend the elbow of the arm on the floor to allow your torso to start dropping toward the floor. As your torso drops, keep it level and don't rotate to one side or the other. This can be adjusted by the degree that you bend the arm on the floor. You should feel a stretch in the area under the arm and along the side torso of the arm on the chair. Hold for the recommended duration, and repeat with the other arm.

Recommended Duration
30 seconds

Modifications
If you are unable to hold yourself with one hand on the chair, place both forearms on the chair. This may decrease the stretch along the sides of your torso, but will increase the extension that occurs in your upper back.

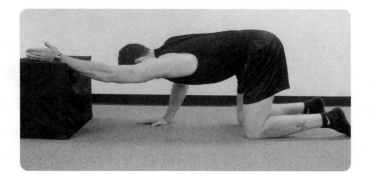

Purpose
To lengthen the muscles from under the arm that attach along the lower back and the pelvis. You should feel the stretch under your arm and along the side of your body.

KNEELING HIP FLEXOR
STRETCH (see page 150)

Begin with one knee on the floor. Keep both legs in line with the hips. The foot of the front leg should be slightly in front of the knee of the same leg. The foot of the back leg should be directly in line with the knee of the back leg. Place your hands on top of the thigh of the front leg and keep your torso straight up and down. Tighten your abdominals and slightly tilt your pelvis backward, decreasing the arch in your lower back. Once you have done this, lunge slightly forward, bringing the front knee over the front ankle. Once in this position, lift the arm on the kneeling side of the body up and over the head for a side stretch. Keep your abdominals tight the entire time. Hold for the recommended duration, then repeat on the other side.

Recommended Duration
1 minute

Modifications
If you are challenged with balance during this exercise, kneel next to a chair and place one hand on the chair to help you maintain your balance. Getting a proper stretch with this exercise is more important than the balance component. If your knee is uncomfortable, place a thin, flat pillow under it during the exercise.

Purpose
To lengthen the hip flexor muscles, which have a significant influence on the lower back. You should feel a stretch in the thigh and the groin of the back leg.

ANKLE SQUEEZES PRONE (see page 147)

Lie on your stomach with your hands on the floor and your chin resting on your hands. Grab hold of a 6- to 8-inch ball or pillow with your ankles. Bend your knees to 90 degrees, holding onto the ball. The 90-degree angle at the knees is a very important part of this exercise. From this position, gently squeeze and release the ball with your inner ankle bones and the inside borders of your feet. Don't squeeze with only the heels.

Recommended Sets and Repetitions
3 sets of 20 repetitions

Modifications
If you don't feel the contraction in your buttocks, spread your knees apart slightly until you do feel the work in the buttocks area. If you feel pressure or pain in your lower back with your knees bent, perform the exercise with your legs straight on the floor.

Purpose
To activate the buttocks muscles and the deep muscles under the buttocks. This improves the relationship of these muscles with the lower back and helps with hip alignment. The contraction should be felt in your buttocks area.

WALL SIT WITH SHOULDER ROTATION

Stand leaning against a wall. Your feet should point straight ahead, directly in line with your hips. Walk your feet out away from the wall. As you walk your feet away, begin sliding your buttocks down the wall. Walk your feet away far enough to allow you to bend your knees close to a 90-degree angle. Press your lower back flat into the wall, and keep the weight on your heels. From this position, get your upper back and head against the wall.

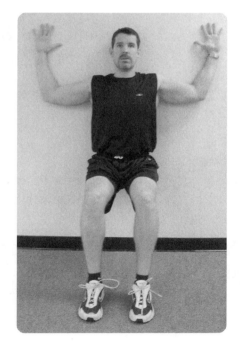

Then place your elbows at shoulder level on the wall. Bend your elbows to 90 degrees, and try to get your upper arms, forearms, wrists, and hands all to touch the wall. Don't allow your lower back to come off the wall. Keep your lower back flat on the wall by using your abdominals. Hold this position for the recommended duration *After you finish*, immediately walk around the room for 20 to 30 seconds to allow the blood to recirculate through your body.

Recommended Duration
30 seconds to 2 minutes, depending on strength

Modifications
You can modify how far you drop your buttocks down the wall. The arms may also be kept below shoulder level, with the hands resting on the thighs, palms-up.

Purposes
To strengthen the thigh muscles and to get the back completely flat on the wall, in order to disengage the lower back muscles. This exercise should be felt in the front thigh muscles.

Program 3.3
Form 3, Category 3 (Multitasker)

ADDUCTOR SQUEEZES IN THE 90-90 NEUTRAL BACK (see page 144)

Lie on your back, with your legs draped over a chair or an ottoman. Place a 6-inch ball or a firm pillow between your knees. Your knees should be in line with your hips. Relax your arms out to the sides, with the palms facing the ceiling. Gently squeeze and release the pillow with your knees. Don't allow your lower back to arch off the floor as you squeeze.

Recommended Sets and Repetitions
3 sets of 15 repetitions

Modifications
None

Purpose
To activate the inner thigh muscles and assist in relaxing the lower back and the buttocks muscles. You should feel this exercise in your inner thighs.

TVA DRAW ON ALL FOURS (see page 145)

Start on your hands and knees with your hands directly under your shoulders and your knees directly under your hips. Your body should be square, like a box. Your weight should be evenly distributed between all four points of contact. Relax your feet so that the tops of the feet rest on the floor. Allow gravity to pull your belly slightly toward the floor. We are trying to achieve a "neutral" spine, which means just a slight arch in the lower back. From this position, draw your belly button to your spine as if you were hollowing out your abdominal area. To use the appropriate muscles for this, you cannot move your spine or hips as you draw in. They should remain still. Once you have drawn all the way in, hold the contraction. You should feel the work toward the lower, inner part of the abdominals. You may even feel it in the deep pelvic floor muscles.

Recommended Duration and Repetitions
Hold for 3 seconds for 10 repetitions. Increase the hold time as you get more comfortable with the exercise.

Modifications
Lie on your back with your knees bent if you are unable to recruit the proper muscles in this exercise or are unable to perform the exercise without moving your hips and spine. Instead, draw your belly button to the floor, again without moving your hips.

Purpose
To assist the body in using the deepest abdominal and "core" muscles for spinal stabilization. These muscles are underused in many people, who instead substitute with the more superficial abdominals.

ONE-ARM TABLE TOP STRETCH
KNEELING (see page 156)

Kneel in front of a chair or a couch. Bend forward and place one hand on the floor under your shoulder and the other forearm on the chair. The elbow of the arm on the chair should be straight, with the thumb pointing to the ceiling. Tighten your abdominals so that your lower back is not arching toward the floor. Bend the elbow of the arm on the floor to allow your torso to start dropping toward the floor. As your torso drops, keep it level and don't rotate to one side or the other. This can be adjusted by the degree that you bend the arm on the floor. You should feel a stretch in the area under the arm and along the side torso of the arm on the chair. Hold for the recommended duration, and repeat with the other arm.

Recommended Duration
30 seconds

Modifications
If you are unable to hold yourself with one hand on the chair, place both forearms on the chair. This may decrease the stretch along the sides of your torso, but it will increase the extension that occurs in your upper back.

Purpose
To lengthen the muscles from under the arm that attach along the lower back and the pelvis. You should feel the stretch under your arm and along the side of your body.

WALL HAMSTRING STRETCH (see page 114)

Lie on your back on the floor next to a wall. Place your legs straight up the wall with your feet, knees, and hips in line. Your body should be perpendicular to the wall. Ideally, your buttocks will be touching the wall. With your legs straight, pull the tops of your feet and toes back toward you. Tighten your front thigh muscles to straighten the knees. The upper buttocks area and the lower back should be resting firmly on the floor. Your arms are relaxed out to the sides, with the palms facing the ceiling. Hold this position for the recommended duration. You should feel a stretch in your calves and the backs of your thighs (hamstrings). Remember, a muscle stretch should not be so intense that it is painful. If this is the case, see the following modification.

Recommended Duration
1 to 1½ minutes

Modification
Move your buttocks away from the wall enough to be able to tolerate the stretch or to allow your upper buttocks and lower back to rest on the floor.

Purpose
To symmetrically lengthen the posterior muscles of the legs without the influence of the spinal muscles. Pulling the feet back and tightening the quadriceps helps to improve the efficiency of the stretch. You should feel the stretch in your calves and the backs of your thighs (hamstrings).

WALL HAMSTRING STRETCH WITH FEMUR ROTATIONS (see page 115)

Lie on your back on the floor next to a wall. Place your legs straight up the wall with your feet about 18 inches apart. Your body should be perpendicular to the wall. Ideally, your buttocks will be touching the wall. With your legs straight, pull the tops of your feet and toes back toward you. Tighten the front thigh muscles to straighten the knees. Your upper buttocks area and lower back should be resting firmly on the floor. Your arms are relaxed out to the sides, with the palms facing the ceiling. From this position, rotate both of your entire legs (not just your feet) toward each other. Then rotate them away from each other. Rotate only as far as you can while keeping the front thigh muscles tight. Think about the entire leg moving as if it were one unit. Continue rotating back and forth in a continuous smooth motion for the recommended repetitions.

Recommended Sets and Repetitions
3 sets of 10 repetitions

Modifications
Move your buttocks away from the wall enough to be able to tolerate the stretch or to allow your upper buttocks and lower back to rest on the floor.

Purpose
To teach the body how to move the hip joints independently of the pelvis. It also strengthens the muscles that rotate the hip in and out. You should feel the movement occurring from around the hip joints. You may feel a slightly different stretch than you felt in the Wall Hamstring Stretch.

KNEELING HIP FLEXOR
STRETCH (see page 150)

Begin with one knee on the floor. Keep both legs in line with the hips. The foot of the front leg should be slightly in front of the knee of the same leg. The foot of the back leg should be directly in line with the knee of the back leg. Place your hands on top of the thigh of the front leg, and keep your torso straight up and down. Tighten your abdominals and slightly tilt your pelvis backward, decreasing the arch in your lower back. Once you have done this, lunge slightly forward, bringing the front knee over the front ankle. Once in this position, lift the arm on the kneeling side of the body up and over the head for a side stretch. Keep your abdominals tight the entire time. Hold for the recommended duration, then repeat on the other side.

Recommended Duration
1 minute

Modifications
If you are challenged with balance during this exercise, kneel next to a chair and place one hand on the chair to help you maintain your balance. Getting a proper stretch with this exercise is more important than the balance component. If your knee is uncomfortable, place a thin, flat pillow under it during the exercise.

Purpose
To lengthen the hip flexor muscles, which have a significant influence on the lower back. You should feel a stretch in the thigh and the groin of the back leg.

SHOULDER BRIDGE WITH ABDOMINALS

Lie on your back with your knees bent. Your feet, knees, and hips are in line, and your feet are pointing straight ahead. Place your arms out to the sides of your body with the lower arms parallel to your head and the palms facing the ceiling. Draw your belly button down to the floor, and tighten all of your abdominal muscles to flatten your lower back entirely to the floor. This serves as the reference point for the position of your pelvis in this exercise. Holding this abdominal position and the tilt to the pelvis that it creates, lift your buttocks off the floor. Your feet and shoulders stay on the ground, while you lift only the buttocks. Keep your knees in line with your hips as you lift, and don't allow them to spread apart. Lift only as high as you can while maintaining this neutral position in your lower back. If you feel your lower back arching, lower your buttocks back toward the floor until you can keep your lower back neutral. Hold for the recommended duration.

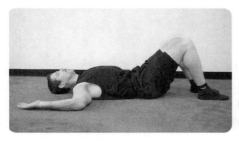

Recommended Sets and Duration
2 sets for 30 seconds each

Modifications
If you are unable to hold for the recommended time, lower your buttocks to the floor and regain the neutral position, then rise back up and hold.

Purpose
This exercise is designed to strengthen the muscles that will assist in bringing your pelvis to a neutral position. You should feel the work in your abdominals, buttocks, and hamstrings (backs of the thighs).

WALL SIT WITH SHOULDER ROTATION (see page 159)

Stand leaning against a wall. Your feet should point straight ahead, directly in line with your hips. Walk your feet out away from the wall. As you walk your feet away, begin sliding your buttocks down the wall. Walk your feet away far enough to allow you to bend your knees close to a 90-degree angle. Press your lower back flat into the wall, and keep the weight on your heels. From this position, get your upper back and head against the wall. Then place your elbows at shoulder level on the wall. Bend your elbows to 90 degrees, and try to get your upper arms, forearms, wrists, and hands all to touch the wall. Don't allow your lower back to come off the wall. Keep your lower back flat on the wall by using your abdominals. Hold this position for the recommended duration. *After you finish*, immediately walk around the room for 20 to 30 seconds to allow the blood to recirculate through your body.

Recommended Duration
30 seconds to 2 minutes, depending on strength

Modifications
You can modify how far you drop your buttocks down the wall. The arms may also be kept below shoulder level, with the hands resting on the thighs, palms-up.

Purposes
To strengthen the thigh muscles and to get the back completely flat on the wall, in order to disengage the lower back muscles. This exercise should be felt in the front thigh muscles.

11

Form 4 Exercises

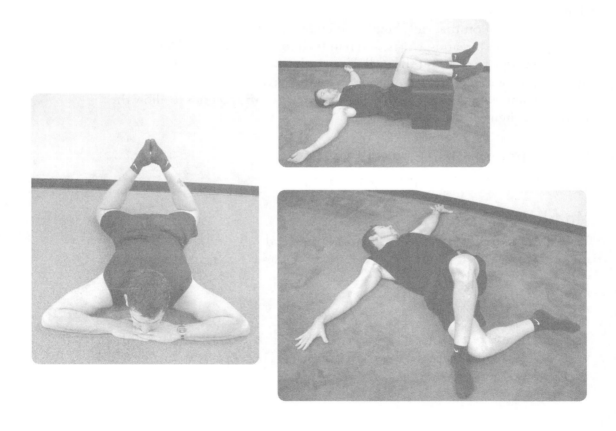

ADDUCTOR SQUEEZES IN THE 90-90 NEUTRAL BACK (see page 144)

Lie on your back, with your legs draped over a chair or an ottoman. Place a 6-inch ball or a firm pillow between your knees. Your knees should be elevated and in line with your hips. Relax your arms out to the sides, with the palms facing the ceiling. Gently squeeze and release the pillow with your knees. Don't allow your lower back to arch off the floor as you squeeze.

Recommended Sets and Repetitions
3 sets of 15 repetitions

Modifications
None

Purpose
To activate the inner thigh muscles and assist in relaxing the lower back and the buttocks muscles. You should feel this exercise in your inner thighs.

ONE-LEGGED HAMSTRING CURLS IN THE 90-90 NEUTRAL BACK

While lying on your back with your lower legs elevated on a chair or a comparable object, slightly point the toes of each foot away from you. One leg at a time, gently press the heel and the back of the calf downward, as if you were trying to bring your heel toward your buttocks. Release and repeat with the opposite leg, alternating each repetition. You should feel this exercise in the calf and the hamstring of the leg that is working. You should also feel a subtle movement of your pelvis on the floor as you press.

Recommended Sets and Repetitions
3 sets of 10 repetitions with each leg

Modifications
None

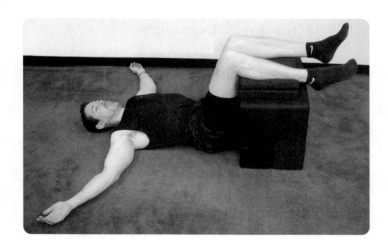

Purpose
To use the leverage of the muscles pushing into the chair to help neutralize the pelvis on the floor.

ANKLE SQUEEZES PRONE (see page 147)

Lie on your stomach with your hands on the floor and your chin resting on your hands. Grab hold of a 6- to 8-inch ball or pillow with your ankles. Bend your knees to 90 degrees, holding onto the ball. The 90-degree angle at the knees is a very important part of this exercise. From this position, gently squeeze and release the ball with your inner ankle bones and the inside borders of your feet. Don't squeeze with only the heels.

Recommended Sets and Repetitions
3 sets of 20 repetitions

Modifications
If you don't feel the contraction in your buttocks, spread your knees apart slightly until you do feel the work in the buttocks area. If you feel pressure or pain in your lower back with your knees bent, perform the exercise with your legs straight on the floor.

Purpose
To activate the buttocks muscles and the deep muscles under the buttocks. This improves the relationship of these muscles with the lower back and helps with hip alignment. The contraction should be felt in your buttocks area.

The next three exercises are done in a sequence. This means that you go through one set of each of the three exercises completely. Then you return to the first exercise and repeat all three exercises a second time. Finally, return to the first exercise and repeat all three for a third time.

ADDUCTOR SQUEEZES SUPINE (see page 95)

Lie on your back with your knees bent. Your feet should point straight ahead and your feet, knees, and hips should be in a straight line. Your arms are out to the sides on the floor, with the palms facing up. Place a 6- to 8-inch ball or pillow between your knees. Gently squeeze and release the pillow with your knees. You should feel this in your inner thighs.

Recommended Sets and Repetitions
3 sets of 20 repetitions

Modifications
None

Purpose
To activate the inner thigh muscles, which are important in pelvic stabilization. They also assist in the inward rotation of the thigh at the hip joint.

ABDUCTOR PRESSES SUPINE (see page 96)

Lie on your back with your knees bent. Your feet should point straight ahead, and your feet, knees, and hips should be in a straight line. Place a non-elastic belt or strap around your thighs, just above the knees. Gently press out and release against the strap as if you were trying to separate your knees. You should feel this in your outer thighs and buttocks.

Recommended Sets and Repetitions
3 sets of 20 repetitions

Modifications
Bring your knees closer together before placing the strap around your thighs to help you feel the exercise in the right muscles.

Purpose
To activate the outer thigh muscles, which are important in pelvic stabilization. They also assist in the outward rotation of the thigh at the hip joint. In addition, this exercise may assist in the positioning of your sacroiliac joint. The exercise should be felt in the outer thighs/hips and the buttocks.

FROG

Lie on your back on the floor. Bring the soles of your feet together, and as you do this, allow your knees to fall out to the sides. Pull your feet toward your groin, making sure that your feet are centered in the middle of your body. Allow gravity to pull your knees toward the floor. Don't try to push your knees down, and don't resist if they drop. Your lower back doesn't have to be flat on the floor, and you shouldn't feel pain in your back.

Recommended Duration
1 minute

Modifications
The degree to which you pull your feet in toward your groin will affect the stretch. The closer your feet are to your groin, the greater the stretch.

Purpose
To lengthen the inner thigh muscles and use their pull to position the pelvis in a symmetrical position. You should feel the stretch in the inner thighs, and your lower back will arch slightly off the floor.

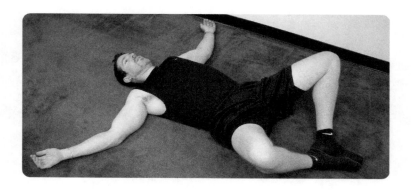

HIP TWIST SUPINE

Lie on your back with your knees bent. Your feet should point straight ahead, and your feet, knees, and hips should be in a straight line. Cross your left ankle over your right knee, and with the muscles of the hip, gently press the left knee away from your body. Your arms are out to your sides at shoulder level, with the palms facing the floor. Using your arms to anchor your upper body in place, begin rolling your hips toward the right. From here, you will slowly lower your left foot flat to the floor on the outside of the right knee. The right knee stays bent while the right leg is flat on the floor. Keep the left knee gently pressed away from the body, with the left foot flat on the floor. Hold this position for the recommended duration. Slowly rise back up, reversing the process. Switch legs, and repeat to the opposite side.

Recommended Duration
1 minute

Modifications
If the stretch is too aggressive, place a book or a pillow on the floor at the area where your foot would land if it went to the floor. Put your foot on the book instead of on the floor to decrease the degree of stretch in the hip area. If the stress on your shoulders is too much, bring your arms down slightly closer to your sides.

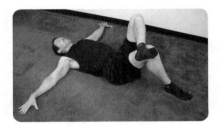

Purpose
To lengthen the outer thigh and hip muscles and introduce some rotation in the hips and the spine. You should feel a stretch in the right outer thigh, the hip, and the lower back area.

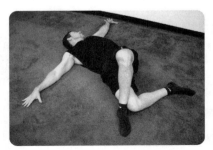

CAT AND DOG (see page 46)

Start on your hands and knees with your hands directly under your shoulders and your knees directly under your hips. Your body should be square, like a box. Your weight should be evenly distributed between all four points of contact. Relax your feet so that the tops of the feet rest on the floor. From this position, smoothly round up your back, draw your belly button toward your spine, and tuck your pelvis under. Drop your head and bring your chin toward your chest. From here, reverse directions by allowing your stomach to drop and your back to sway. Your shoulder blades should drop together and your head looks up. Make it one fluid movement rather than holding any one position. Exhale as your head looks up, and inhale as your head looks down. It's important to keep your elbows straight as you perform the movement and to avoid rocking forward and backward at the hips and the shoulders.

Recommended Repetitions
15 repetitions

Modifications
You can limit the range of motion in either or both directions if you feel any restrictions or discomfort during the exercise.

Purpose
To improve motion of the entire spine, in both flexion and extension. It also provides a gentle stretch of the spinal flexors and extensors and helps with coordinating movement of the head and the pelvis.

176   THE PAIN-FREE PROGRAM

ADDUCTOR SQUEEZES IN THE 90-90 NEUTRAL BACK (see page 144)

Lie on your back, with your legs draped over a chair or an ottoman. Place a 6-inch ball or a firm pillow between your knees. Your knees should be elevated and in line with your hips. Relax your arms out to the sides, with the palms facing the ceiling. Gently squeeze and release the pillow with your knees. Don't allow your lower back to arch off the floor as you squeeze.

Recommended Sets and Repetitions

3 sets of 15 repetitions

Modifications

None

Purpose

To activate the inner thigh muscles and assist in relaxing the lower back and the buttocks muscles. You should feel this exercise in your inner thighs.

ANKLE SQUEEZES PRONE (see page 147)

Lie on your stomach with your hands on the floor and your chin resting on your hands. Grab hold of a 6- to 8-inch ball or pillow with your ankles. Bend your knees to 90 degrees, holding onto the ball. The 90-degree angle at the knees is a very important part of this exercise. From this position, gently squeeze and release the ball with your inner ankle bones and the inside borders of your feet. Don't squeeze with only the heels.

Recommended Sets and Repetitions
3 sets of 20 repetitions

Modifications
If you don't feel the contraction in your buttocks, spread your knees apart slightly until you do feel the work in the buttocks area. If you feel pressure or pain in your lower back with your knees bent, perform the exercise with your legs straight on the floor.

Purpose
To activate the buttocks muscles and the deep muscles under the buttocks. This improves the relationship of these muscles with the lower back and helps with hip alignment. The contraction should be felt in your buttocks area.

WALL HAMSTRING STRETCH (see page 114)

Lie on your back on the floor next to a wall. Place your legs straight up the wall with your feet, knees, and hips in line. Your body should be perpendicular to the wall. Ideally, your buttocks will be touching the wall. With your legs straight, pull the tops of your feet and toes back toward you. Tighten your front thigh muscles to straighten the knees. The upper buttocks area and the lower back should be resting firmly on the floor. Your arms are relaxed out to the sides with the palms facing the ceiling. Hold this position for the recommended duration. You should feel a stretch in your calves and the backs of your thighs (hamstrings). Remember, a muscle stretch should not be so intense that it is painful. If this is the case, see the following modification.

Recommended Duration
1 to 1½ minutes

Modification
Move your buttocks away from the wall enough to be able to tolerate the stretch or to allow your upper buttocks and lower back to rest on the floor.

Purpose
To symmetrically lengthen the posterior muscles of the legs without the influence of the spinal muscles. Pulling the feet back and tightening the quadriceps helps to improve the efficiency of the stretch. You should feel the stretch in your calves and the backs of your thighs (hamstrings).

WALL HAMSTRING STRETCH WITH FEMUR ROTATIONS (see page 115)

Lie on your back on the floor next to a wall. Place your legs straight up the wall with your feet about 18 inches apart. Your body should be perpendicular to the wall. Ideally, your buttocks will be touching the wall. With your legs straight, pull the tops of your feet and toes back toward you. Tighten the front thigh muscles to straighten the knees. Your upper buttocks area and lower back should be resting firmly on the floor. Your arms are relaxed out to the sides, with the palms facing the ceiling. From this position, rotate both of your entire legs (not just your feet) toward each other. Then rotate them away from each other. Rotate only as far as you can while keeping the front thigh muscles tight. Think about the entire leg moving as if it were one unit. Continue rotating back and forth in a continuous smooth motion for the recommended repetitions.

Recommended Sets and Repetitions
3 sets of 10 repetitions

Modifications
Move your buttocks away from the wall enough to be able to tolerate the stretch or to allow your upper buttocks and lower back to rest on the floor.

Purpose
To teach the body how to move the hip joints independently of the pelvis. It also strengthens the muscles that rotate the hip in and out. You should feel the movement occurring from around the hip joints. You may feel a slightly different stretch than you felt in the Wall Hamstring Stretch.

OPPOSITE ARM AND LEG GLIDING (see page 122)

Lie face down on the floor. Place a small folded towel or a washcloth under your forehead to keep your face off the floor. Lie with your arms straight out above your head and your legs in line with your hips. From this position, you will attempt to lengthen your body on opposite sides by reaching in a direct line with your body along the floor with one arm and in the opposite direction with the opposite leg. Hold this position for 5 seconds and relax. Repeat the movement with the other arm and leg. For each repetition, alternate the sides that you are reaching with. While you reach, it's very important that you remain in contact with the floor. Don't lift your arms or your hips as you reach. Imagine that you are moving on a sheet of ice. You should feel a stretch on the side of the lower back of the leg that is reaching, as well as muscular contraction around your upper back and the shoulder of the arm that is reaching.

Recommended Repetitions and Duration
Hold for 5 seconds for 10 repetitions on each side, alternating sides on each repetition.

Modifications
If you experience discomfort in your shoulder, reach on a slight angle away from the body, instead of in a direct line with the body.

Purpose
To work the small, intrinsic muscles that stabilize the spine. This exercise also requires reciprocal movement of the upper and the lower body, similar to walking.

KNEELING HIP FLEXOR
STRETCH (see page 150)

Begin with one knee on the floor. Keep both legs in line with the hips. The foot of the front leg should be slightly in front of the knee of the same leg. The foot of the back leg should be directly in line with the knee of the back leg. Place your hands on top of the thigh of the front leg, and keep your torso straight up and down. Tighten your abdominals and slightly tilt your pelvis backward, decreasing the arch in your lower back. Once you have done this, lunge slightly forward, bringing the front knee over the front ankle. Once in this position, lift the arm on the kneeling side of the body up and over the head for a side stretch. Keep your abdominals tight the entire time. Hold for the recommended duration, then repeat on the other side.

Recommended Duration
1 minute

Modifications
If you are challenged with balance during this exercise, kneel next to a chair and place one hand on the chair to help you maintain your balance. Getting a proper stretch with this exercise is more important than the balance component. If your knee is uncomfortable, place a thin, flat pillow under it during the exercise.

Purpose
To lengthen the hip flexor muscles, which have a significant influence on the lower back. You should feel a stretch in the thigh and the groin of the back leg.

TABLE TOP WALL STRETCH (see page 126)

Stand facing a wall with your feet, knees, and hips all in alignment. Stand a little more than an arm's length away from the wall. Lean forward and reach out, placing the palms of your hands on the wall at approximately shoulder height. Straighten your elbows. Kick your buttocks backward, and allow your torso to drop down between your arms. You should bend from the hip joints and move your torso down between your arms as a unit. This should increase the arch in your back. Tighten your quadriceps (front thighs), and hold for the desired length of time.

Recommended Duration
1 minute

Modifications
Place your hands higher up on the wall and limit the distance you drop your torso down between your arms.

Purpose
To lengthen the muscles on the back side of the leg while shortening the muscles of the back. Your arms on the wall assist in keeping your back in extension while the backs of your thighs lengthen. You should feel the stretch in your hamstrings (back of the thighs) and calves. You may also feel a stretch alongside your torso and a tightening in the upper back.

Program 4.3
Form 4, Category 3 (Multitasker)

ADDUCTOR SQUEEZES IN THE 90-90 NEUTRAL BACK (see page 144)

Lie on your back, with your legs draped over a chair or an ottoman. Place a 6-inch ball or a firm pillow between your knees. Your knees should be elevated and in line with your hips. Relax your arms out to the sides, with the palms facing the ceiling. Gently squeeze and release the pillow with your knees. Don't allow your lower back to arch off the floor as you squeeze.

Recommended Sets and Repetitions
3 sets of 15 repetitions

Modifications
None

Purpose
To activate the inner thigh muscles and assist in relaxing the lower back and the buttocks muscles. You should feel this exercise in your inner thighs.

ANKLE SQUEEZES PRONE (see page 147)

Lie on your stomach with your hands on the floor and your chin resting on your hands. Grab hold of a 6- to 8-inch ball or pillow with your ankles. Bend your knees to 90 degrees, holding on to the ball. The 90-degree angle at the knees is a very important part of this exercise. From this position, gently squeeze and release the ball with your inner ankle bones and the inside borders of your feet. Don't squeeze with only the heels.

Recommended Sets and Repetitions
3 sets of 20 repetitions

Modifications
If you don't feel the contraction in the buttocks, spread your knees apart slightly until you do feel the work in the buttocks area. If you feel pressure or pain in your lower back with your knees bent, perform the exercise with your legs straight on the floor.

Purpose
To activate the buttocks muscles and the deep muscles under the buttocks. This improves the relationship of these muscles with the lower back and helps with hip alignment. The contraction should be felt in your buttocks area.

ACTIVE FROG PRONE

Lie on your stomach with your hands on the floor and your chin resting on your hands. Walk your feet apart as far as you can, spreading the legs as far apart as possible. From here, bend your knees and place the soles of your feet together. Be sure to line up your feet evenly, with the balls of the feet and the heels of both feet touching each other. Next, gently press and release the soles of the feet into one another. Make certain to press equally with both the heels and the balls of the feet.

Recommended Sets and Repetitions
3 sets of 20 repetitions

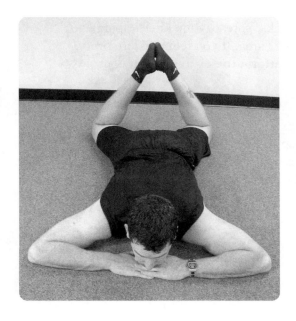

Modifications
None

Purpose
To strengthen the outward rotator muscles of the hips and the buttocks. You should feel this exercise in your upper, inner thighs and buttocks.

SWAY-BACK ANKLE SQUEEZES (see page 125)

Kneel on the floor. Place an approximately 6-inch pillow or ball between your ankles. Drop forward so that you are on your hands and knees. If viewed from the side, your hip joints should be slightly ahead of the knee joints and your shoulders should be directly over the hands. Your fingers should point straight ahead. Relax your abdominal muscles, and allow your back to drop into a sway-back position. Keep your elbows straight. Allow your head to hang down. Gently squeeze and release the pillow between your ankles, using the inner ankle bones and the inside borders of the feet. You should feel a contraction around your hips and buttocks. Continue for the desired number of sets and repetitions. When resting between sets, rest only from the squeezing; maintain the sway-back position while you rest from the squeezing.

Recommended Sets and Repetitions
3 sets of 20 repetitions

Modifications
This exercise can be modified in two ways. The first would be to back the hips up over the knees to relieve some of the pressure from the lower back. The second would be to rest on the forearms with the elbows bent. The elbows, instead of the hands, would then be directly under the shoulders.

Purpose
To strengthen the muscles of the hips while the lower back is in a position of passive extension. You should feel a contraction around the hips and the buttocks.

OPPOSITE ARM AND LEG GLIDING (see page 122)

Lie face down on the floor. Place a small folded towel or a washcloth under your forehead to keep your face off the floor. Lie with your arms straight out above your head and your legs in line with your hips. From this position, you will attempt to lengthen your body on opposite sides by reaching in a direct line with your body along the floor with one arm and in the opposite direction with the opposite leg. Hold this position for 5 seconds and relax. Repeat the movement with the other arm and leg. For each repetition, alternate the sides that you are reaching with. While you reach, it's very important that you remain in contact with the floor. Don't lift your arms or your hips as you reach. Imagine that you are moving on a sheet of ice. You should feel a stretch on the side of the lower back of the leg that is reaching, as well as muscular contraction around your upper back and the shoulder of the arm that is reaching.

Recommended Repetitions and Duration
Hold for 5 seconds for 10 repetitions on each side, alternating sides on each repetition.

Modifications
If you experience discomfort in your shoulder, reach on a slight angle away from the body, instead of in a direct line with the body.

Purpose
To work the small, intrinsic muscles that stabilize the spine. This exercise also requires reciprocal movement of the upper and the lower body, similar to walking.

HIP TWIST SUPINE (see page 175)

Lie on your back with your knees bent. Your feet should point straight ahead, and your feet, knees, and hips should be in a straight line. Cross your left ankle over your right knee, and with the muscles of the hip, gently press the left knee away from your body. Your arms are out to your sides at shoulder level, with the palms facing the floor. Using your arms to anchor your upper body in place, begin rolling your hips toward the right. From here, you will slowly lower your left foot flat to the floor on the outside of the right knee. The right knee stays bent while the right leg is flat on the floor. Keep the left knee gently pressed away from your body, with the left foot flat on the floor. Hold this position for the recommended duration. Slowly rise back up, reversing the process. Switch legs, and repeat to the opposite side.

Recommended Duration
1 minute

Modifications
If the stretch is too aggressive, place a book or a pillow on the floor at the area where your foot would land if it went to the floor. Place your foot on the book instead of on the floor to decrease the degree of stretch in the hip area. If the stress on your shoulders is too much, bring your arms down slightly closer to your sides.

Purpose
To lengthen the outer thigh and hip muscles and introduce some rotation in the hips and the spine. You should feel a stretch in the right outer thigh, the hip, and the lower back area.

CAT AND DOG (see page 46)

Start on your hands and knees with your hands directly under your shoulders and your knees directly under your hips. Your body should be square, like a box. Your weight should be evenly distributed between all four points of contact. Relax your feet so that the tops of the feet rest on the floor. From this position, smoothly round up your back, draw your belly button toward your spine, and tuck your pelvis under. Drop your head and bring your chin toward your chest. From here, reverse directions by allowing your stomach to drop and your back to sway. Your shoulder blades should drop together and your head looks up. Make it one fluid movement, rather than holding any one position. Exhale as your head looks up, and inhale as your head looks down. It's important to keep your elbows straight as you perform the movement and to avoid rocking forward and backward at the hips and the shoulders.

Recommended Repetitions
15 repetitions

Modifications
You can limit the range of motion in either or both directions if you feel any restrictions or discomfort during the exercise.

Purpose
To improve motion of the entire spine, in both flexion and extension. It also provides a gentle stretch of the spinal flexors and extensors and helps with coordinating movement of the head and the pelvis.

WALL HAMSTRING STRETCH WITH FEMUR ROTATIONS (see page 115)

Lie on your back on the floor next to a wall. Place your legs straight up the wall with your feet about 18 inches apart. Your body should be perpendicular to the wall. Ideally, your buttocks will be touching the wall. With your legs straight, pull the tops of your feet and toes back toward you. Tighten the front thigh muscles to straighten the knees. Your upper buttocks area and lower back should be resting firmly on the floor. Your arms are relaxed out to the sides, with the palms facing the ceiling. From this position, rotate both of your entire legs (not just your feet) toward each other. Then rotate them away from each other. Rotate only as far as you can while keeping the front thigh muscles tight. Think about the entire leg moving as if it were one unit. Continue rotating back and forth in a continuous smooth motion for the recommended repetitions.

Recommended Sets and Repetitions
3 sets of 10 repetitions

Modifications
Move your buttocks away from the wall enough to be able to tolerate the stretch or to allow your upper buttocks and lower back to rest on the floor.

Purpose
To teach the body how to move the hip joints independently of the pelvis. It also strengthens the muscles that rotate the hip in and out. You should feel the movement occurring from around the hip joints. You may feel a slightly different stretch than you felt in the Wall Hamstring Stretch.

12

Form 5 Exercises

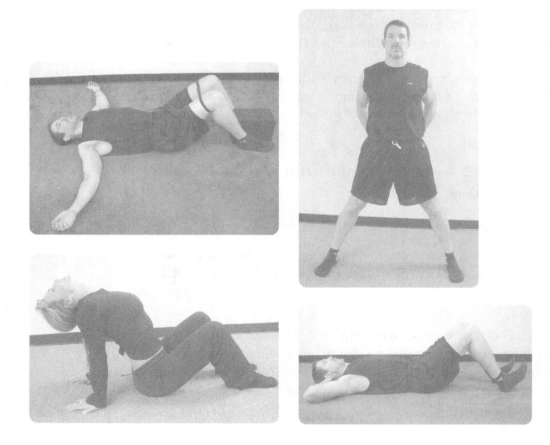

PULLOVERS IN THE 90-90 NEUTRAL BACK POSITION

Lie on your back, with your legs draped over a chair or an ottoman. Reach your arms straight out above your chest. Clasp your hands together and keep the elbows straight. From this position, bring your clasped hands overhead toward the floor behind you. Go only as far back as you can while keeping your elbows straight. If your elbows bend, stop at that point and return to the start. Repeat the overhead movement, using a slow, controlled motion. You should feel an increase in the arch throughout your back as your hands draw closer to the floor. You may also feel some muscular effort around the shoulder joints. Repeat for the recommended sets and repetitions.

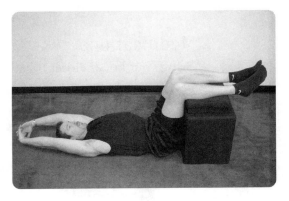

Recommended Sets and Repetitions
3 sets of 10 repetitions

Modifications
If there is any discomfort or limitation in the shoulder joints, keep the movement of the arms in a pain-free range.

Purpose
To focus the effort on the muscles of the upper spine and improve the position of the shoulder joints in relation to the upper back without the assistance of the lower back.

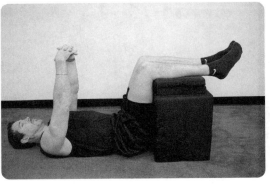

ABDUCTOR PRESSES IN THE 90-90 NEUTRAL BACK POSITION

In this exercise, your knees are slightly closer together than your hips and ankles. Lie on your back, with your legs draped over a chair or an ottoman. Place a non-elastic belt or strap around your thighs, just above the knees, and elevate your lower legs. Gently press out and release against the strap, as if you were trying to separate your knees. You should feel this in your outer thighs and buttocks.

Recommended Sets and Repetitions
3 sets of 15 repetitions

Modifications
Bring your knees closer together or farther apart to help you feel the exercise in the right muscles.

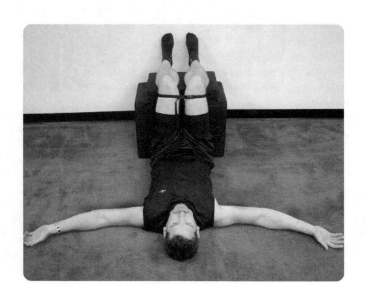

Purpose
To activate the outer thigh muscles without using the lower back muscles. The outer thigh muscles are important in pelvic stabilization and the outward rotation of the thigh at the hip joint. This exercise may also assist in the positioning of your sacroiliac joint. The exercise should be felt in the outer thighs/hips and the buttocks.

FROG (see page 174)

Lie on your back on the floor. Bring the soles of your feet together, and as you do this, allow your knees to fall out to the sides. Pull your feet toward your groin, making sure that your feet are centered in the middle of your body. Allow gravity to pull your knees toward the floor. Don't try to push your knees down and don't resist if they drop. Your lower back doesn't have to be flat on the floor, and you shouldn't feel pain in your back.

Recommended Duration
1 minute

Modifications
The degree to which you pull your feet in toward your groin will affect the stretch. The closer your feet are to your groin, the greater the stretch.

Purpose
To lengthen the inner thigh muscles and use their pull to position the pelvis in a symmetrical position. You should feel the stretch in the inner thighs, and your lower back will arch slightly off the floor.

HIP TWIST SUPINE (see page 175)

Lie on your back with your knees bent. Your feet should point straight ahead, and your feet, knees, and hips should be in a straight line. Cross your left ankle over your right knee, and with the muscles of the hip, gently press the left knee away from your body. Your arms are out to your sides at shoulder level, with the palms facing the floor. Using your arms to anchor your upper body in place, begin rolling your hips toward the right. From here, you will slowly lower your left foot flat to the floor on the outside of the right knee. The right knee stays bent while the right leg is flat on the floor. Keep the left knee gently pressed away from the body, with the left foot flat on the floor. Hold this position for the recommended duration. Slowly rise back up, reversing the process. Switch legs, and repeat to the opposite side.

Recommended Duration
1 minute

Modifications
If the stretch is too aggressive, place a book or a pillow on the floor at the area where your foot would land if it went to the floor. Put your foot on the book instead of on the floor to decrease the degree of stretch in the hip area. If the stress on your shoulders is too much, bring your arms down slightly closer to your sides.

Purpose
To lengthen the outer thigh and hip muscles and introduce some rotation in the hips and the spine. You should feel a stretch in the right outer thigh, the hip, and the lower back area.

CAT AND DOG (see page 46)

Start on your hands and knees with your hands directly under your shoulders and your knees directly under your hips. Your body should be square, like a box. Your weight should be evenly distributed between all four points of contact. Relax your feet so that the tops of the feet rest on the floor. From this position, smoothly round up your back, draw your belly button toward your spine, and tuck your pelvis under. Drop your head and bring your chin toward your chest. From here, reverse directions by allowing your stomach to drop and your back to sway. Your shoulder blades should drop together and your head looks up. Make it one fluid movement, rather than holding any one position. Exhale as your head looks up, and inhale as your head looks down. It's important to keep your elbows straight as you perform the movement and to avoid rocking forward and backward at the hips and the shoulders.

Recommended Repetitions
15 repetitions

Modifications
You can limit the range of motion in either or both directions if you feel any restrictions or discomfort during the exercise.

Purpose
To improve motion of the entire spine, in both flexion and extension. It also provides a gentle stretch of the spinal flexors and extensors and helps with coordinating movement of the head and the pelvis.

TABLE TOP WALL STRETCH (see page 126)

Stand facing a wall with your feet, knees, and hips all in alignment. Stand a little more than an arm's length away from the wall. Lean forward and reach out, placing the palms of your hands on the wall at approximately shoulder height. Straighten your elbows. Kick your buttocks backward, and allow your torso to drop down between your arms. You should bend from the hip joints and move your torso down between your arms as a unit. This should increase the arch in your back. Tighten your quadriceps (front thighs) and hold for the desired length of time.

Recommended Duration
1 minute

Modifications
Place your hands higher up on the wall and limit the distance you drop your torso down between your arms.

Purpose
To lengthen the muscles on the back side of the leg, while shortening the muscles of the back. Your arms on the wall assist in keeping your back in extension while the backs of the thighs lengthen. You should feel the stretch in your hamstrings (back of the thighs) and calves. You may also feel a stretch alongside your torso and a tightening in the upper back.

HEEL DROP ON STAIRS (see page 100)

Stand at the bottom of a stairwell or in a doorway with a platform compara-ble to the height of a single stair, with the balls of your feet on the step. Your feet should be about 4 to 6 inches apart and pointing straight ahead. Place one hand on the nearest handrail, or stand in the middle and use both handrails if possible. Allow your heels to drop down. As you do this, it's very important that you keep your body aligned straight up and down, if viewed from the side. Imagine a straight line extending from your ear to your shoulder to your hip to your knee to your ankle. Don't bend forward at the waist, and don't allow your hips to move ahead of the rest of your body.

Recommended Duration

2 to 3 minutes

Modifications

To increase or decrease the amount of stretch in your calves, get more or less of your foot on the step.

Purpose

Although you'll feel an obvious stretch in your calves, this isn't the primary purpose of the exercise. By keeping the body aligned perfectly, as described, you are using many of your postural muscles to maintain and "learn" this position.

Program 5.2
Form 5, Category 2 (Dexterity Work)

SNOW ANGELS IN 90-90
NEUTRAL BACK (see page 103)

Lie on your back, with your legs draped over a chair or an ottoman. Rest your arms on the floor at your sides. Keep your fingers, wrists, and elbows straight. The little-finger-side of the hand will be the only part of the hand to touch the floor. Raise your arms along the floor, with your elbows straight up to shoulder level. At shoulder level, rotate your entire arm and hand back so that the thumb-side of the hand is touching the floor. From this position, bring your hands along the floor and overhead, keeping your elbows straight. Reverse the process on the way down. Lower your arms with the thumb-side on the floor until they're shoulder level. Rotate your arms forward so that the little-finger-side of the hand is on the floor, then return them along your sides and repeat.

Recommended Sets and Repetitions
3 sets of 10 repetitions

Modifications
Limit how far overhead you go with your hands if you have to bend your elbows. Alternately, you may continue the overhead movement until your palms touching as long as your elbows remain straight.

Purpose
First, to assist the body in recruiting the muscles that extend the upper back. In addition, to teach the body to coordinate the movement of the arm with the shoulder blade. You should feel the muscles of your shoulders and upper and middle back working. You may feel a stretch along your arms.

DOUBLE-ARM DOORWAY STRETCH (see page 119)

Stand in a doorjamb with one foot inside the doorjamb and one foot outside of it. Place the palms of your hands and your forearms on the doorjamb so that your elbows are bent to 90 degrees. The upper arms should be level with the shoulders. Tighten your abdominal muscles. Keep your chest high, and avoid shrugging your shoulders. Then lean your upper body through the doorjamb until you feel the stretch in your chest area. Hold this position for the recommended duration. After your first hold, relax, then switch the front and the back foot placement and repeat.

Recommended Sets and Duration
2 sets of 30 seconds

Modifications
Slightly vary the height of the elbow position to change the emphasis of the area stretched or to relieve any discomfort in the shoulders.

Purpose
To lengthen the muscles of the chest and the front shoulders, which will help to "open" the chest area. The stretch should be felt across your chest and front shoulders.

UPPER SPINAL ROTATION (see page 105)

Lie on your side in the fetal position, with your hips and knees bent to 90 degrees. Your ankles, knees, hips, and shoulders should be stacked directly over one another. Place your bottom arm straight out on the floor at 90 degrees from your torso, and place the top hand on top of the bottom hand. From this position, rotate your top hand off your bottom hand toward the floor behind you. It's very important that you keep your knees together as you rotate. Let the weight of your top arm pull your body around. It's crucial to breathe, relax, and allow gravity to slowly bring your arm toward the floor. Your head should be relaxed on the floor, and your eyes should face the ceiling. After the desired time, slowly return to the starting position and repeat with the other side.

Recommended Duration

1 to 2 minutes

Modifications

If you have trouble keeping your knees together, reach down with your bottom hand to help hold your knees in place.

Purpose

To improve the spine's ability to rotate independently of the hips and the pelvis. You should feel a stretch across your chest and the top arm and a stretch along the side of your body and toward the lower back.

CAT AND DOG (see page 46)

Start on your hands and knees with your hands directly under your shoulders and your knees directly under your hips. Your body should be square, like a box. Your weight should be evenly distributed between all four points of contact. Relax your feet so that the tops of the feet rest on the floor. From this position, smoothly round up your back, draw your belly button toward your spine, and tuck your pelvis under. Drop your head and bring your chin toward your chest. From here, reverse directions by allowing your stomach to drop and your back to sway. Your shoulder blades should drop together and your head looks up. Make it one fluid movement, rather than holding any one position. Exhale as your head looks up, and inhale as your head looks down. It's important to keep your elbows straight as you perform the movement and to avoid rocking forward and backward at the hips and shoulders.

Recommended Repetitions
15 repetitions

Modifications
You can limit the range of motion in either or both directions if you feel any restrictions or discomfort during the exercise.

Purpose
To improve motion of the entire spine, in both flexion and extension. It also provides a gentle stretch of the spinal flexors and extensors and helps with coordinating movement of the head and the pelvis.

TABLE TOP WALL STRETCH (see page 126)

Stand facing a wall with your feet, knees, and hips all in alignment. Stand a little more than an arm's length away from the wall. Lean forward and reach out, placing the palms of your hands on the wall at approximately shoulder height. Straighten your elbows. Kick your buttocks backward, and allow your torso to drop down between your arms. You should bend from the hip joints and move your torso down between your arms as a unit. This should increase the arch in your back. Tighten your quadriceps (front thighs), and hold for the desired length of time.

Recommended Duration
1 minute

Modifications
Place your hands higher up on the wall and limit the distance you drop your torso down between your arms.

Purpose
To lengthen the muscles on the back side of the leg while shortening the muscles of the back. Your arms on the wall assist in keeping your back in extension while the backs of the thighs lengthen. You should feel the stretch in your hamstrings (back of the thighs) and calves. You may also feel a stretch along-side your torso and a tightening in the upper back.

SITTING THORACIC AND CERVICAL EXTENSION

Sit on the floor with your knees bent and your feet flat on the floor. Place your hands behind you for support with the fingers pointing away from your body. Your elbows should be straight. Roll your hips forward with help from your arms to create an arch in your lower back. Lift your chest up and out, using your upper/middle back muscles. Allow your head to drop back as if you were staring at the ceiling. Try to relax your head back as far as it will go. Avoid shrugging your shoulders up around your ears. You may feel a "bunching" in the back of your neck. This is okay. You should not feel pain. Hold this position for the recommended duration.

Recommended Sets and Duration
2 sets of 30 seconds

Modifications
If your neck is painful, continue with the proper positioning of your upper and lower back. Move your head into a pain-free area, and focus your eyes toward the ceiling.

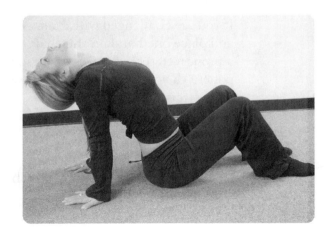

Purpose
To strengthen the muscles of the middle back and lengthen the muscles on the front of the neck. You should feel the muscular effort in your middle back, lifting your chest up and out, and a stretch on the front of your neck.

KNEELING HIP FLEXOR
STRETCH (see page 150)

Begin with one knee on the floor. Keep both legs in line with the hips. The foot of the front leg should be slightly in front of the knee of the same leg. The foot of the back leg should be directly in line with the knee of the back leg. Place your hands on top of the thigh of the front leg, and keep your torso straight up and down. Tighten your abdominals and slightly tilt your pelvis backward, decreasing the arch in your lower back. Once you have done this, lunge slightly forward, bringing the front knee over the front ankle. Once in this position, lift the arm of the kneeling side of the body up and over the head for a side stretch. Keep your abdominals tight the entire time. Hold for the recommended duration, then repeat on the other side.

Recommended Duration
1 minute

Modifications
If you are challenged with balance during this exercise, kneel next to a chair and place one hand on the chair to help you maintain your balance. Getting a proper stretch with this exercise is more important than the balance component. If your knee is uncomfortable, place a thin, flat pillow under it during the exercise.

Purpose
To lengthen the hip flexor muscles, which have a significant influence on the lower back. You should feel a stretch in the thigh and the groin of the back leg.

WALL HAMSTRING STRETCH (see page 114)

Lie on your back on the floor next to a wall. Place your legs straight up the wall with your feet, knees, and hips in line. Your body should be perpendicular to the wall. Ideally, your buttocks will be touching the wall. With your legs straight, pull the tops of your feet and toes back toward you. Tighten your front thigh muscles to straighten the knees. The upper buttocks area and the lower back should be resting firmly on the floor. Your arms are relaxed out to the sides, with the palms facing the ceiling. Hold this position for the recommended duration. You should feel a stretch in your calves and the backs of your thighs (hamstrings). Pulling the feet back and tightening the quadriceps helps to improve the efficiency of the stretch. Remember, a muscle stretch should not be so intense that it is painful. If this is the case, see the following modification.

Recommended Duration
1 minute to 1½ minutes

Modification
Move your buttocks away from the wall enough to be able to tolerate the stretch or to allow your upper buttocks and lower back to rest on the floor.

Purpose
To symmetrically lengthen the posterior muscles of the legs without the influence of the spinal muscles.

PULLOVERS IN THE 90-90 NEUTRAL BACK POSITION (see page 193)

Lie on your back, with your legs draped over a chair or an ottoman. Reach your arms straight out above your chest. Clasp your hands together and keep the elbows straight. From this position, bring your clasped hands overhead toward the floor behind you. Go only as far back as you can while keeping your elbows straight. If your elbows bend, stop at that point and return to the start. Repeat the overhead movement, using a slow, controlled motion. You should feel an increase in the arch throughout your back as your hands draw closer to the floor. You may also feel some muscular effort around the shoulder joints. Repeat for the recommended sets and repetitions.

Recommended Sets and Repetitions
3 sets of 10 repetitions

Modifications
If there is any discomfort or limitation in the shoulder joints, keep the movement of the arms in a pain-free range.

Purpose
To focus the effort on the muscles of the upper spine and improve the position of the shoulder joints in relation to the upper back without the assistance of the lower back.

ISO ABDUCTION ADDUCTION SUPINE

Lie on your back with your knees bent. Your feet should point straight ahead, and your feet, knees, and hips should be in a straight line. Place a 6- to 8-inch pillow or block between your ankles. Put a non-elastic belt or strap around your thighs, just above the knees. Your arms are out to the sides, with the palms facing the ceiling. Gently press out and release against the strap as if you were trying to separate your knees. *At the same time*, press in against the pillow as if you were trying to slide your feet together. Release and repeat for the recommended sets and repetitions. Be careful not to turn the bottoms of your feet onto the pillow as you push or to lift the heels off the ground as you push. You should feel this in your inner and outer thighs and buttocks.

Recommended Sets and Repetitions
3 sets of 10 repetitions

Modifications
None

Purpose
To help reposition the hip joint by strengthening the muscles around it.

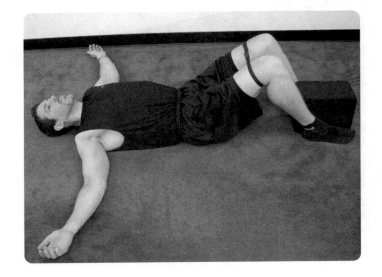

ISO ADDUCTION ABDUCTION SUPINE

Lie on your back with your knees bent. Your feet should point straight ahead, and your feet, knees, and hips should be in a straight line. Place a 6- to 8-inch pillow or block between your knees. Place a non-elastic belt or strap around your ankles. Your arms are out to the sides, with the palms facing the ceiling. Gently press on the pillow with your knees. *At the same time*, press out against the strap as if you were trying to slide your feet apart. You should feel this in your inner and outer thighs and buttocks. Release and repeat for the recommended sets and repetitions.

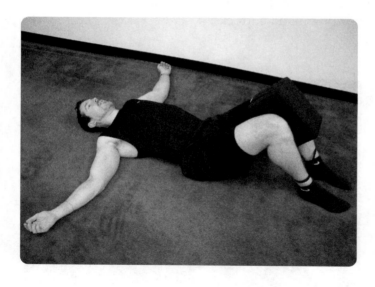

Recommended Sets and Repetitions
3 sets of 10 repetitions

Modifications
None

Purpose
To help reposition the hip joint by strengthening the muscles around it.

HIP TWIST SUPINE (see page 175)

Lie on your back with your knees bent. Your feet should point straight ahead, and your feet, knees, and hips should be in a straight line. Cross your left ankle over your right knee, and with the muscles of the hip, gently press the left knee away from your body. Your arms are out to your sides at shoulder level, with the palms facing the floor. Using your arms to anchor your upper body in place, begin rolling your hips toward the right. From here, you will slowly lower the left foot flat to the floor on the outside of the right knee. The right knee stays bent, while the right leg is flat on the floor. Keep the left knee gently pressed away from your body, with the left foot flat on the floor. Hold this position for the recommended duration. Slowly rise back up, reversing the process. Switch legs, and repeat to the opposite side.

Recommended Duration
1 minute

Modifications
If the stretch is too aggressive, place a book or a pillow on the floor at the area where your foot would land if it went to the floor. Put your foot on the book instead of on the floor to decrease the degree of stretch in the hip area. If the stress on your shoulders is too much, bring your arms down slightly closer to your sides.

Purpose
To lengthen the outer thigh and hip muscles and introduce some rotation in the hips and the spine. You should feel a stretch in the right outer thigh, the hip, and the lower back area.

CAT AND DOG (see page 46)

Start on your hands and knees with your hands directly under your shoulders and your knees directly under your hips. Your body should be square, like a box. Your weight should be evenly distributed between all four points of contact. Relax your feet so that the tops of the feet rest on the floor. From this position, smoothly round up your back, draw your belly button toward your spine, and tuck your pelvis under. Drop your head and bring your chin toward your chest. From here, reverse directions by allowing your stomach to drop and your back to sway. Your shoulder blades should drop together and your head looks up. Make it one fluid movement, rather than holding any one position. Exhale as your head looks up, and inhale as your head looks down. It's important to keep your elbows straight as you perform the movement and to avoid rocking forward and backward at the hips and the shoulders.

Recommended Repetitions
15 repetitions

Modifications
You can limit the range of motion in either or both directions if you feel any restrictions or discomfort during the exercise.

Purpose
To improve motion of the entire spine, in both flexion and extension. It also provides a gentle stretch of the spinal flexors and extensors and helps with coordinating movement of the head and the pelvis.

ABDOMINAL CRUNCHES WITH HEELS

Lie on your back with your knees bent. Your feet should point straight ahead and your feet, knees, and hips should be in a straight line. Slightly lift the front of your feet and toes off the floor. Keep the pressure down and toward you with your heels into the floor. This should make you engage the muscles on the backs of your thighs (hamstrings). Flatten your lower back into the floor, using your abdominal muscles. Interlock your fingers behind your head, and focus on the ceiling above you. Rise up, using your abdominals, until your shoulder blades lift off the floor. Exhale on your way up, and inhale on the way back down. Remember to keep the pressure on the floor with your heels so that you feel the backs of your thighs working. Lower and repeat for the recommended sets and repetitions.

Recommended Sets and Repetitions
3 sets of 10 repetitions

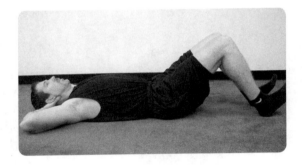

Modifications
If the exercise is too challenging with your hands behind your head, place your hands on your thighs. Reach for the tops of your knees by lifting your shoulder blades off the ground.

Purpose
To teach your body to work and strengthen your abdominal muscles without using your hip flexor muscles. You should feel this in both your upper and lower abdominal areas.

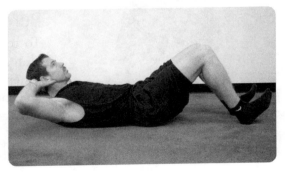

SPREAD-FOOT GLUTEAL CONTRACTIONS

While standing, spread your legs apart until you feel a very slight stretch in your inner thigh muscles. Your feet should be pointing straight ahead. Your knees should be in a "soft extension," which means that they should be straight but not locked. From this position, squeeze and release the buttocks muscles. Focus on isolating the buttocks muscles and not using the quadriceps (thighs) or the abdominals. It can be helpful during this exercise to place your hands on your buttocks while you squeeze. The tactile information from your hands can help you to recruit the right muscles.

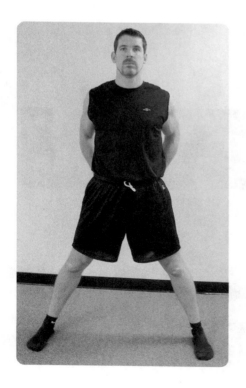

Recommended Sets and Repetitions
3 sets of 20 repetitions

Modifications
If you have difficulty engaging your buttocks muscles at first, try turning your feet out until you can feel that you are using the right muscles. Once you have done that, return your feet to pointing straight ahead.

Purpose
To teach your body to recruit the very important gluteal muscles while standing, without using the inner thigh or the hamstring muscles. You should feel the entire buttocks muscles contract when you squeeze and not just the small, deep muscles of the anus.

STANDING HIP HINGE (see page 141)

Stand with your feet hip-width apart and pointing straight ahead. Place your hands on your hips so that the thumbs are to the front over the hip bones and pointing down. The rest of your fingers should be resting on the upper buttocks and pointing toward the floor. Try to squeeze your elbows together and hold. Tighten your front thigh muscles. Keeping an arch in the lower back, bend forward and hinge from the hip joints. Bend only as far forward as you can without losing the arch in your lower back. Shift the weight toward the balls of your feet, and focus your eyes straight ahead. Hold for the recommended duration. You should feel a stretch in your calves and hamstrings. You may also feel the muscular effort in your lower back.

Recommended Duration
45 seconds to 1 minute

Modifications
Instead of placing your hands on your lower back, stand in front of a dining table or a desk and place your hands on that. Use your upper body to control how far you bend forward. It's still critical that you maintain the arch in your lower back and hinge from the hip as you lean forward.

Purpose
To lengthen the hamstring and the calf muscles against gravity, while stabilizing the lumbar spine with the spinal extensor muscles.

13

Form 6 Exercises

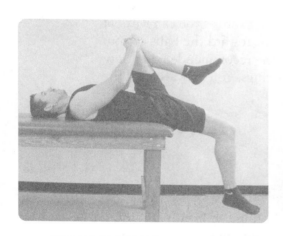

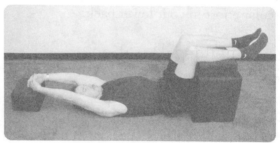

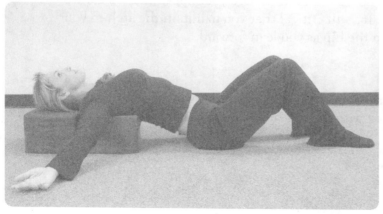

Program 6.1

REVERSE BENCH PRESS IN 90-90 NEUTRAL BACK (see page 94)

Lie on your back, with your legs draped over a chair or an ottoman. Place your arms on the floor, at shoulder level. Bend your elbows to 90 degrees so that your wrists are directly over the elbows. Your hands are open, with the palms of your hands facing forward. From this position, gently press and release your elbows into the floor. This should cause your shoulder blades to come together. Do this without shrugging your shoulders.

Recommended Sets and Repetitions
3 sets of 15 repetitions

Modifications
If you feel this exercise in your neck, slightly lower your elbows toward your sides, to avoid using the neck muscles.

Purpose
To activate the muscles between the shoulder blades and the muscles of the middle/upper back. This assists in bringing the shoulders back to a more anatomically correct position.

PULLOVER PRESSES IN THE 90-90 NEUTRAL BACK POSITION

Place a 6- to 10-inch stack of pillows or books on the floor about 8 inches from the top of your head. Lie on your back, with your legs draped over a chair or an ottoman. Reach your arms straight out above your chest. Clasp your hands together and keep the elbows straight. From this position, bring your clasped hands overhead toward the floor behind you until your hands reach the stack of books. Be sure that the height of the books allows you to keep your elbows straight when your hands are on top. If you cannot keep your elbows straight, add more books until you can. With your hands resting on the book stack, gently press and release your clasped hands into the stack as if you were trying to continue moving toward the floor, but the books are in the way. You should feel your shoulder blades move together and an increase in the arch throughout your back as you press. You may also feel some muscular effort around your shoulder joints. Repeat for the recommended sets and repetitions.

Recommended Sets and Repetitions
3 sets of 10 repetitions

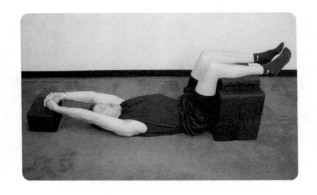

Modifications
If there is any discomfort or limitation in the shoulder joints, raise the height of the book stack until you can press pain-free with your elbows straight.

Purpose
To strengthen the muscles of your upper back and shoulders by using your arms to help your body recruit the muscles of your upper back.

TVA DRAW ON ALL FOURS (see page 145)

Start on your hands and knees with your hands directly under your shoulders and your knees directly under your hips. Your body should be square, like a box. Your weight should be evenly distributed between all four points of contact. Relax your feet so that the tops of the feet rest on the floor. Allow gravity to pull your belly slightly toward the floor. We are trying to achieve a "neutral" spine, which means just a slight arch in the lower back. From this position, draw your belly button to your spine as if you were hollowing out your abdominal area. To use the appropriate muscles for this, you cannot move your spine or hips as you draw in. They should remain still. Once you have drawn all the way in, hold the contraction. You should feel the work toward the lower, inner part of the abdominals. You may even feel it in the deep pelvic floor muscles.

Recommended Duration and Repetitions
Hold for 3 seconds for 10 repetitions. Increase the hold time as you get more comfortable with the exercise.

Modifications
Lie on your back with your knees bent if you are unable to recruit the proper muscles in this exercise or are unable to perform the exercise without moving your hips and spine. Instead, draw your belly button to the floor, again without moving your hips.

Purpose
To assist the body in using the deepest abdominal and "core" muscles for spinal stabilization. These muscles are underused in many people, who instead substitute with the more superficial abdominals.

QUADRICEPS STRETCH
STANDING (see page 154)

Stand facing the back of a chair at an arm's length away. Place a chair or an object with a comparable height and surface behind you. Stand with your feet pointing straight ahead and your feet directly under your hips. Place the top of one foot on the back or the arm of the chair. The height of your foot place-ment determines how much stretch you feel in your front thigh muscles. When you first put your foot up on the chair, you should be aware of a mild stretch. Once you've got your foot on the chair, you must adjust your alignment. Make sure that both knees are aligned side to side. One should not be in front of the other. Place your hands on the chair in front of you to keep your torso straight up and down. From this position, you will rotate your pelvis posteriorly (tip the punch bowl backward). When you rotate your pelvis, you should feel an increase in the stretch in your front thigh muscles. Be careful not to push the pelvis forward instead of rotating the pelvis backward.

Recommended Duration
1 minute

Modifications
The height that the foot is propped up behind you dictates the stretch. Increase the height of your foot with a pillow to increase the stretch.

Purpose
To lengthen the quadriceps muscles and position the pelvis in neutral. This stretch should be felt from the knee to the front of the hip.

HIP FLEXOR STRETCH ON TABLE

Sit on the edge of a countertop or a table. The surface should be high enough so that your feet don't touch the ground. Lie all the way back on the table, while keeping your knees bent to 90 degrees. Your buttocks should be close to the edge of the table. Bring one knee to your chest, and place one hand behind that knee and the other hand on top of the knee. Allow the other leg to drop straight down off the table. The muscle tension on the leg hanging down will cause your back to arch. Use your abdominals to keep your lower back flat on the table. Hold for the recommended duration. Switch legs, and repeat with the other side.

Recommended Duration
1 to 1½ minutes

Modifications
If the stretch is too great in the front groin and thigh, or if you are unable to keep your lower back flat on the table, move slightly up on the table so that more of the thigh that is level with your torso is supported.

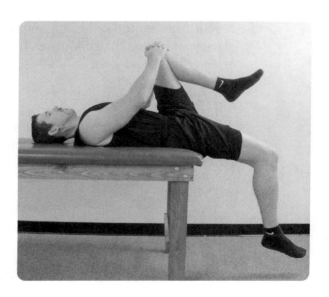

Purpose
To passively lengthen the hip flexor muscles and strengthen control of the abdominal muscles on the pelvis. You should feel a stretch in the front thigh and the groin of the leg hanging down.

HIP ROTATOR STRETCH (see page 98)

Lie on your back with your feet flat on a wall and your knees and hips bent to a 90-degree angle. Cross the left ankle over the right knee. As you do this, it's extremely important that your hips stay square to the wall. The tendency is for the pelvis to rotate away if the hips are tight. Using the muscles of your right hip (not your hand), gently press the right knee away from your body toward the wall. Remember to keep your hips square on the floor. Hold this position for the desired amount of time. You should feel the stretch in the area of the right buttocks. Repeat with the opposite leg.

Recommended Duration
1 to 2 minutes

Modifications
If your hips are too tight and you cannot keep your hips square to the wall, place your feet on the floor instead of on the wall. Perform the stretch the same as described previously.

Purpose
To assist in positioning the hip joint by elongating the deep outward rotators of the hip. This stretch should be felt in the buttocks of the leg with the ankle crossed.

THORACIC BLOCK WITH HEAD SUPPORTED

Prepare two 8-inch stacks of books or very firm pillows. Place them end to end. Sit on the floor with your back to the end of one stack. Your buttocks should be about 12 inches from the books. Keep your knees bent. Lie back onto the stack so that the closest edge to you lines up just below your shoulder blades. The first stack of books should support your upper back, and the

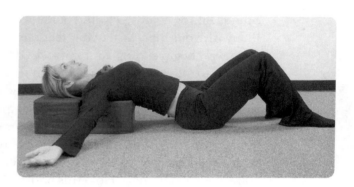

second stack should support your head. Your arms are out to the sides at shoulder level, with the palms facing the ceiling. Try to relax and settle into this position for the recommended duration.

Recommended Duration
2 to 3 minutes

Modifications
If your head is unable to reach the second stack that should support it, slightly increase the height of that stack. However, you don't want the stack so high that it pushes your head forward.

Purpose
This position will help to passively improve the extension in your upper back and will decrease the rounding. You should feel an "opening" of the chest and the front of the shoulders. You may feel a little pressure in your middle back.

WALL SIT WITH SHOULDER ROTATION (see page 159)

Stand leaning against a wall. Your feet should point straight ahead, directly in line with your hips. Walk your feet out away from the wall. As you walk your feet away, begin sliding your buttocks down the wall. Walk your feet away far enough to allow you to bend your knees close to a 90-degree angle. Press your lower back flat into the wall, and keep the weight on your heels. From this position, get your upper back and head against the wall. Then place your elbows at shoulder level on the wall. Bend your elbows to 90 degrees, and try to get your upper arms, forearms, wrists, and hands all to touch the wall. Don't allow your lower back to come off the wall. Keep your lower back flat on the wall by using your abdominals. Hold this position for the recommended duration. *After you finish*, immediately walk around the room for 20 to 30 seconds to allow the blood to recirculate through your body.

Recommended Duration
30 seconds to 2 minutes, depending on strength

Modifications
You can modify how far you drop your buttocks down the wall. The arms may also be kept below shoulder level with the hands resting on the thighs, palms-up.

Purpose
To strengthen the thigh muscles and to get your back completely flat on the wall, in order to disengage the lower back muscles. Placing the arms on the wall strengthens the muscles of the upper back and the shoulders and causes the abdominals to work harder. This exercise should be felt in the front thigh muscles, the upper back, and the abdominals.

REVERSE BENCH PRESS IN 90-90 NEUTRAL BACK (see page 94)

Lie on your back, with your legs draped over a chair or an ottoman. Place your arms on the floor, at shoulder level. Bend your elbows to 90 degrees so that your wrists are directly over the elbows. Your hands are open, with the palms of the hands facing forward. From this position, gently press and release your elbows into the floor. This should cause your shoulder blades to come together. Do this without shrugging your shoulders.

Recommended Sets and Repetitions
3 sets of 15 repetitions

Modifications
If you feel this exercise in your neck, slightly lower your elbows toward your sides, to avoid using the neck muscles.

Purpose
To activate the muscles between the shoulder blades and the muscles of the middle/upper back. This assists in bringing the shoulders back to a more anatomically correct position.

PULLOVER PRESSES IN THE 90-90 NEUTRAL BACK POSITION (see page 218)

Place a 6- to 10-inch stack of pillows or books on the floor about 8 inches from the top of your head. Lie on your back, with your legs draped over a chair or an ottoman. Reach your arms straight out above your chest. Clasp your hands together and keep the elbows straight. From this position, bring your clasped hands overhead toward the floor behind you until your hands reach the stack of books. Be sure that the height of the books allows you to keep your elbows straight when your hands are on top. If you cannot keep your elbows straight, add more books until you can. With your hands resting on the book stack, gently press and release your clasped hands into the stack as if you were trying to continue moving toward the floor, but the books are in the way. You should feel your shoulder blades move together and an increase in the arch throughout your back as you press. You may also feel some muscular effort around your shoulder joints. Repeat for the recommended sets and repetitions.

Recommended Sets and Repetitions
3 sets of 10 repetitions

Modifications
If there is any discomfort or limitation in the shoulder joints, raise the height of the book stack until you can press pain-free with your elbows straight.

Purpose
To strengthen the muscles of your upper back and shoulders by using your arms to help your body recruit the muscles of your upper back.

DOUBLE-ARM DOORWAY STRETCH (see page 119)

Stand in a doorjamb with one foot inside the doorjamb and one foot outside of it. Place the palms of your hands and your forearms on the doorjamb so that your elbows are bent to 90 degrees. The upper arms should be level with the shoulders. Tighten your abdominal muscles. Keep your chest high and avoid shrugging your shoulders. Then lean your upper body through the doorjamb until you feel the stretch in your chest area. Hold this position for the recommended duration. After your first hold, relax; then switch the front and the back foot placement and repeat.

Recommended Sets and Duration
2 sets of 30 seconds

Modifications
Slightly vary the height of the elbow position to change the emphasis of the area stretched or to relieve any discomfort in the shoulders.

Purpose
To lengthen the muscles of the chest and the front shoulders, which will help to "open" the chest area. The stretch should be felt across your chest and front shoulders.

ONE-ARM TABLE TOP STRETCH
KNEELING (see page 156)

Kneel in front of a chair or a couch. Bend forward and place one hand on the ground under your shoulder and the other forearm on the chair. The elbow of the arm on the chair should be straight with the thumb pointing to the ceiling. Tighten your abdominals so that your lower back is not arching toward the floor. Bend the elbow of the arm on the floor to allow your torso to start dropping toward the floor. As your torso drops, keep it level and don't rotate to one side or the other. This can be adjusted by the degree that you bend the arm on the floor. You should feel a stretch in the area under the arm and along the side torso of the arm on the chair. Hold for the recommended duration, and repeat with the other arm.

Recommended Duration
30 seconds

Modifications
If you're unable to hold yourself with one hand on the chair, place both forearms on the chair. This may decrease the stretch along the sides of your torso, but it will increase the extension that occurs in your upper back.

Purpose
To lengthen the muscles from under the arm that attach along the lower back and the pelvis. You should feel the stretch under your arm and along the side of your body.

KNEELING HIP FLEXOR STRETCH (see page 150)

Begin with one knee on the floor. Keep both legs in line with the hips. The foot of the front leg should be slightly in front of the knee of the same leg. The foot of the back leg should be directly in line with the knee of the back leg. Place your hands on top of the thigh of the front leg, and keep your torso straight up and down. Tighten your abdominals and slightly tilt your pelvis backward, decreasing the arch in your lower back. Once you have done this, lunge slightly forward, bringing the front knee over the front ankle. Once in this position, lift the arm on the kneeling side of the body up and over the head for a side stretch. Keep your abdominals tight the entire time. Hold for the recommended duration, then repeat on the other side.

Recommended Duration
1 minute

Modifications
If you are challenged with balance during this exercise, kneel next to a chair and place one hand on the chair to help you maintain your balance. Getting a proper stretch with this exercise is more important than the balance component. If your knee is uncomfortable, place a thin, flat pillow under it during the exercise.

Purpose
To lengthen the hip flexor muscles, which have a significant influence on the lower back. You should feel a stretch in the thigh and the groin of the back leg.

ANKLE SQUEEZES KNEELING WITH ABDOMINAL HOLD (see page 151)

Kneel upright on the floor with your knees directly under your hips. The tops of your feet are flat on the floor. Place a 6- to 8-inch ball or pillow between your ankles. Allow your arms to hang at your sides. Tighten your abdominals to tilt your pelvis posteriorly. This should decrease the arch in your lower back. Gently squeeze and release the ball with your inner ankle bones and the inside borders of your feet. Don't squeeze with only the heels. The contraction should be felt in your buttocks area.

Recommended Sets and Repetitions
3 sets of 20 repetitions

Modifications
If you don't feel the contraction in your buttocks, spread your knees apart slightly until you do feel the work in the buttocks area. If you are challenged by holding yourself in this position, kneel in front of a chair and support yourself with the seat of the chair. Try to progress from using the chair for balance to balancing on your own.

Purpose
To activate the gluteal muscles and the abdominal muscles and help them to keep the pelvis neutral during upright balance.

WALL HAMSTRING STRETCH (see page 114)

Lie on your back on the floor next to a wall. Place your legs straight up the wall with your feet, knees, and hips in line. Your body should be perpendicular to the wall. Ideally, your buttocks will be touching the wall. With your legs straight, pull the tops of your feet and toes back toward you. Tighten your front thigh muscles to straighten the knees. The upper buttocks area and the lower back should be resting firmly on the floor. Your arms are relaxed out to the sides, with the palms facing the ceiling. Hold this position for the recommended duration. You should feel a stretch in your calves and the backs of your thighs (hamstrings). Remember, a muscle stretch should not be so intense that it is painful. If this is the case, see the following modification.

Recommended Duration
1 to 1½ minutes

Modification
Move your buttocks away from the wall enough to be able to tolerate the stretch or to allow your upper buttocks and lower back to rest on the floor.

Purpose
To symmetrically lengthen the posterior muscles of the legs without the influence of the spinal muscles. Pulling the feet back and tightening the quadriceps helps to improve the efficiency of the stretch. You should feel the stretch in your calves and the backs of your thighs (hamstrings).

WALL SIT WITH SHOULDER ROTATION (see page 159)

Stand leaning against a wall. Your feet should point straight ahead, directly in line with your hips. Walk your feet out away from the wall. As you do this, begin sliding your buttocks down the wall. Walk your feet away far enough to allow you to bend your knees close to a 90-degree angle. Press your lower back flat into the wall and keep the weight on your heels. From this position, get your upper back and head against the wall. Then place your elbows at shoulder level on the wall. Bend your elbows to 90 degrees, and try to get your upper arms, forearms, wrists, and hands all to touch the wall. Don't allow your lower back to come off the wall. Keep your lower back flat on the wall by using your abdominals. Hold this position for the recommended duration. *After you finish*, immediately walk around the room for 20 to 30 seconds to allow the blood to recirculate through your body.

Recommended Duration
30 seconds to 2 minutes, depending on strength

Modifications
You can modify how far you drop your buttocks down the wall. The arms may also be kept below shoulder level with the hands resting on the thighs, palms-up.

Purpose
To strengthen the thigh muscles and to get your back completely flat on the wall, in order to disengage the lower back muscles. Placing your arms on the wall strengthens the muscles of the upper back and the shoulders and causes the abdominals to work harder. This exercise should be felt in the front thigh muscles, the upper back and the abdominals.

REVERSE BENCH PRESS IN 90-90 NEUTRAL BACK (see page 94)

Lie on your back, with your legs draped over a chair or an ottoman. Place your arms on the floor, at shoulder level. Bend your elbows to 90 degrees so that the wrists are directly over the elbows. Your hands are open, with the palms of the hands facing forward. From this position, gently press and release your elbows into the floor. This should cause your shoulder blades to come together. Do this without shrugging your shoulders.

Recommended Sets and Repetitions
3 sets of 15 repetitions

Modifications
If you feel this exercise in your neck, slightly lower your elbows toward your sides, to avoid using the neck muscles.

Purpose
To activate the muscles between the shoulder blades and the muscles of the middle/upper back. This assists in bringing the shoulders back to a more anatomically correct position.

PULLOVER PRESSES IN THE 90-90 NEUTRAL BACK POSITION (see page 218)

Place a 6- to 10-inch stack of pillows or books on the floor about 8 inches from the top of your head. Lie on your back, with your legs draped over a chair or an ottoman. Reach your arms straight out above your chest. Clasp your hands together, and keep the elbows straight. From this position, bring your clasped hands overhead toward the floor behind you until your hands reach the stack of books. Be sure that the height of the books allows you to keep your elbows straight when your hands are on top. If you cannot keep your elbows straight, add more books until you can. With your hands resting on the book stack, gently press and release your clasped hands into the stack as if you were trying to continue moving toward the floor, but the books are in the way. You should feel your shoulder blades move together and an increase in the arch throughout your back as you press. You may also feel some muscular effort around your shoulder joints. Repeat for the recommended sets and repetitions.

Recommended Sets and Repetitions
3 sets of 10 repetitions

Modifications
If there is any discomfort or limitation in the shoulder joints, raise the height of the book stack until you can press pain-free with your elbows straight.

Purpose
To strengthen the muscles of your upper back and shoulders by using your arms to help your body recruit the muscles of your upper back.

UPPER SPINAL ROTATION (see page 105)

Lie on your side in the fetal position, with your hips and knees bent to 90 degrees. Your ankles, knees, hips, and shoulders should be stacked directly over one another. Place your bottom arm straight out on the floor at 90 degrees from your torso, and place the top hand on top of the bottom hand. From this position, rotate your top hand off your bottom hand toward the floor behind you. It's very important that you keep your knees together as you rotate. Let the weight of your top arm pull your body around. It's crucial to breathe, relax, and allow gravity to slowly bring your arm toward the floor. Your head should be relaxed on the floor, and your eyes should face the ceiling. After the desired time, slowly return to the starting position and repeat with the other side.

Recommended Duration
1 to 2 minutes

Modifications
If you have trouble keeping your knees together, reach down with your bottom hand to help hold your knees in place.

Purpose
To improve the spine's ability to rotate independently of the hips and the pelvis. You should feel a stretch across your chest and the top arm and a stretch along the side of your body and toward the lower back.

CAT AND DOG (see page 46)

Start on your hands and knees with your hands directly under your shoulders and your knees directly under your hips. Your body should be square, like a box. Your weight should be evenly distributed between all four points of contact. Relax your feet so that the tops of the feet rest on the floor. From this position, smoothly round up your back, draw your belly button toward your spine, and tuck your pelvis under. Drop your head and bring your chin toward your chest. From here, reverse directions by allowing your stomach to drop and your back to sway. Your shoulder blades should drop together and your head looks up. Make it one fluid movement, rather than holding any one position. Exhale as your head looks up, and inhale as your head looks down. It's important to keep your elbows straight as you perform the movement and to avoid rocking forward and backward at the hips and shoulders.

Recommended Repetitions
15 repetitions

Modifications
You can limit the range of motion in either or both directions if you feel any restrictions or discomfort during the exercise.

Purpose
To improve motion of the entire spine, in both flexion and extension. It also provides a gentle stretch of the spinal flexors and extensors and helps with coordination of movement of the head and the pelvis.

KNEELING HIP FLEXOR
STRETCH (see page 150)

Begin with one knee on the floor. Keep both legs in line with the hips. The foot of the front leg should be slightly in front of the knee of the same leg. The foot of the back leg should be directly in line with the knee of the back leg. Place your hands on top of the thigh of the front leg, and keep your torso straight up and down. Tighten your abdominals and slightly tilt your pelvis backward, decreasing the arch in your lower back. Once you have done this, lunge slightly forward, bringing the front knee over the front ankle. Once in this position, lift the arm on the kneeling side of the body up and over the head for a side stretch. Keep your abdominals tight the entire time. Hold for the recommended duration, then repeat on the other side.

Recommended Duration
1 minute

Modifications
If you are challenged with balance during this exercise, kneel next to a chair and place one hand on the chair to help you maintain your balance. Getting a proper stretch with this exercise is more important than the balance component. If your knee is uncomfortable, place a thin, flat pillow under it during the exercise.

Purpose
To lengthen the hip flexor muscles, which have a significant influence on the lower back. You should feel a stretch in the thigh and the groin of the back leg.

ANKLE SQUEEZES PRONE (see page 147)

Lie on your stomach with your hands on the floor and your chin resting on your hands. Grab hold of a 6- to 8-inch ball or pillow with your ankles. Bend your knees to 90 degrees, holding onto the ball. The 90-degree angle at the knees is a very important part of this exercise. From this position, gently squeeze and release the ball with your inner ankle bones and the inside borders of your feet. Don't squeeze with only the heels.

Recommended Sets and Repetitions
3 sets of 20 repetitions

Modifications
If you don't feel the contraction in your buttocks, spread your knees apart slightly until you do feel the work in the buttocks area. If you feel pressure or pain in your lower back with your knees bent, perform the exercise with your legs straight on the floor.

Purpose
To activate the buttocks muscles and the deep muscles under the buttocks. This improves the relationship of these muscles to the lower back and helps with hip alignment. The contraction should be felt in your buttocks area.

THORACIC BLOCK WITH HEAD SUPPORTED (see page 223)

Prepare two 8-inch stacks of books or very firm pillows. Place them end to end. Sit on the floor with your back to the end of one stack. Your buttocks should be about 12 inches from the books. Keep your knees bent. Lie back on the stack so that the closest edge to you lines up just below your shoulder blades. The first stack of books should support your upper back, and the second stack should support your head. Your arms are out to the sides at shoulder level, with the palms facing the ceiling. Try to relax and settle into this position for the recommended duration.

Recommended Duration
2 to 3 minutes

Modifications
If your head is unable to reach the second stack that should support it, slightly increase the height of that stack. However, you don't want the stack so high that it pushes your head forward.

Purpose
This position will help to passively improve the extension in your upper back and decrease the rounding. You should feel an "opening" of the chest and the front of the shoulders. You may feel a little pressure in your middle back.

SHOULDER BRIDGE WITH ABDOMINALS (see page 166)

Lie on your back with your knees bent. Your feet, knees, and hips are in line, and your feet are pointing straight ahead. Place your arms out to the sides of your body, with the lower arms parallel to your head and the palms facing the ceiling. Draw your belly button down to the floor, and tighten all of your abdominal muscles to flatten your lower back entirely to the floor. This serves as the reference point for the position of your pelvis in this exercise. Holding this abdominal position and the tilt to the pelvis that it creates, lift your buttocks off the floor. Your feet and shoulders stay on the ground, while you lift only the buttocks. Keep your knees in line with your hips as you lift, and don't allow them to spread apart. Lift only as high as you can while maintaining this neutral position in your lower back. If you feel your lower back arching, lower your buttocks back toward the floor until you can keep your lower back neutral. Hold for the recommended duration.

Recommended Sets and Duration
2 sets for 30 seconds each

Modifications
If you are unable to hold for the recommended time, lower your buttocks to the floor and regain the neutral position, then rise back up and hold.

Purpose
This exercise is designed to strengthen the muscles that will assist in bringing your pelvis to a neutral position. You should feel the work in your abdominals, buttocks, and hamstrings (backs of the thighs).

14

The "Graduate" Program

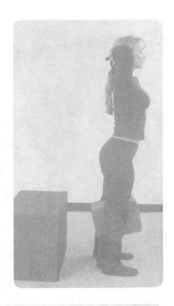

A s stated earlier, the Graduate Program is more advanced and requires greater overall muscular strength and coordination. The ability to do these exercises correctly and to be sure that you are not compensating is dependent on your mastery of the exercises in your personal Form and Category. Don't proceed with these exercises if you're still experiencing significant symptoms. If you've made it to the Graduate Program, congratulations! You've made major progress toward taking control of your health, improving your function, and providing a healing environment for your body to operate in.

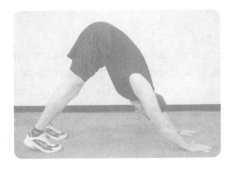

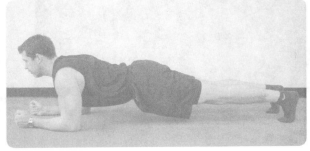

HIP ROTATIONS SUPINE

Lie on your back with your knees bent. Your feet, knees, and hips are in line, and your feet are pointing straight ahead. Place a 6- to 8-inch pillow or ball between the knees. Put your arms out to the sides of your body, with the palms facing the floor. Lift your feet off the floor so that your knees and hips are bent

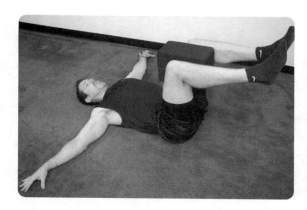

to 90 degrees. In a controlled motion, rotate your legs approximately halfway to the floor on one side of your body. Reverse directions, and bring your legs halfway to the floor on the other side of your body. Keep your upper body anchored in place on the floor with your arms. Be sure to keep the knee and the hip joint angle at 90 degrees as you move.

Recommended Sets and Repetitions
2 sets of 15 repetitions to each side

Modifications
None

Purpose
Strengthening the oblique abdominals as they lengthen to help control gravitational forces. You should feel this exercise in the lower abdominals and along the sides of your torso.

SINGLE-ARM SHOULDER FLEXION

Lie facedown on the floor with one arm straight out on the floor overhead and in line with the body. Keep this arm perfectly straight, and rotate the thumb toward the ceiling by rotating the entire arm from the shoulder. The other arm is relaxed at the side. Draw your belly button toward the spine to hollow your abdominal area, which will help stabilize your body. From this position, lift the arm extended overhead off the floor while keeping the elbow straight. After the desired repetitions, move the same arm to a 45-degree angle from your body and continue to rotate out from the shoulder. Lift and lower from the floor here, while keeping the elbow straight. Finally, move your arm to a 90-degree angle from your body and continue to rotate out from the shoulder. Once again, lift and lower the arm from the floor, keeping the elbow straight.

Recommended Sets and Repetitions
2 sets of 10 repetitions with each arm

Modifications
Don't focus on how high your arm is lifted from the ground. Even if you aren't able to lift the arm, your body will still be strengthening the correct muscles.

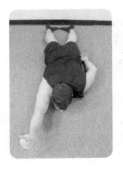
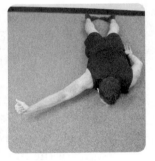
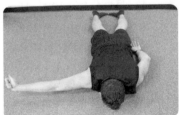

Purpose
To strengthen the muscles of the upper back and the shoulders and to improve their working relationship. You should feel this in the shoulder that you're lifting and in the muscles of the upper back.

HIP ROTATOR STRETCH (UNASSISTED) (see page 98)

This is the same exercise as the Hip Rotator Stretch, but it's done without the help of a wall to support your leg. Lie on your back with your feet flat on the ground and your knees and hips bent. Cross the left ankle over the right knee. Using only the muscles of the hip, lift your right leg off the floor so that the hip and the knee are bent to a 90-degree angle. Using the muscles of your left hip (not your hand), gently press the left knee away from your body. Remember to keep your hips square on the floor. Hold this position for the desired amount of time. Repeat with the opposite leg.

Recommended Duration
1 minute per leg

Modifications
The only modification at this level would be to decrease the time of the exercise.

Purpose
To assist in positioning the hip joint by elongating the deep outward rotators of the hip. It also strengthens the hip flexor of the leg supporting the crossed leg. You should feel this stretch in the buttocks of the leg that has the crossed ankle. You may also feel the effort in your abdominals and the front thigh muscles of the support leg.

SINGLE-LEG SQUATS

Stand with your feet pointing straight ahead. Shift your weight to one leg, and balance on that foot. Using the balance leg, lower your body down in a squat. Make sure that your knee tracks directly in line with your first and second toe as you squat down. Don't allow the knee to rotate or shift toward the other leg. If this happens, limit the depth of the squat. Try to stay balanced on one foot the entire time by not putting your other foot down on the floor. Repeat, and then alternate sets with other leg.

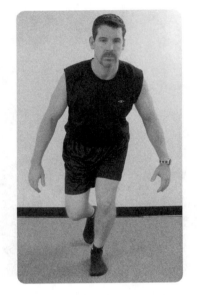

Recommended Sets and Repetitions
3 sets of 5 repetitions per leg

Modifications
If balance is a problem, limit the depth of the squat to a level where you can stay stable.

Purpose
Addresses balance and strength of the important links from the foot and the ankle to the knee, and then to the hip and the lower back. You should feel the work predominantly in the thigh muscles but may also feel it in the shin and calf muscles.

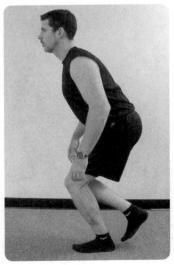

SITTING TO STANDING

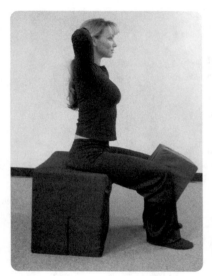

Sit on a firm chair that allows you to have your knees and hips bent to 90 degrees. Sit toward the front of the chair as if it didn't have a backrest. Your feet should point straight ahead, and your feet, knees, and hips should be in a straight line. Roll your pelvis forward, and sit tall on your "sit bones" under the buttocks. This should create an arch in your lower back. Place a 6- to 8-inch ball or pillow between your knees. Interlock your fingers behind your head, and hold the elbows back. Without moving your feet on the floor, rise up to a standing position. Keep your feet and knees in alignment at all times. Stand all the way until your knees are straight. Maintaining the arch in your lower back and without moving your feet, sit back down on the chair. Continue for the recommended sets and repetitions.

Recommended Sets and Repetitions
3 sets of 10 repetitions

Modifications
A chair that allows you to sit with your knees and hips at an angle that's greater than 90 degrees will make the exercise less challenging.

Purpose
To strengthen the muscles of the hips and the pelvis, as well as of the upper back. You should feel this in your thighs and buttocks.

COBRA UP

Lie on your stomach, resting on your elbows and forearms. Your elbows should be directly under the shoulders. Your hands should be in fists. Your feet are in line with your hips. Lifting from the forearms and the hips, raise your body up, keeping your body in line from shoulder to ankle. Relax completely between the shoulder blades and allow them to collapse together so that your upper back is not rounded. Keep the front thigh muscles tight. Don't let your hips drop to the floor. Keep the abdominals engaged to limit the lower back from arching. Keep your eyes focused straight ahead. Hold for the desired time and relax. Repeat the process for the recommended sets and repetitions.

Recommended Sets and Duration
2 sets of 1-minute holds

Modifications
Can be done with the knees still on the floor.

Purpose
To strengthen the core stabilizers of the body.

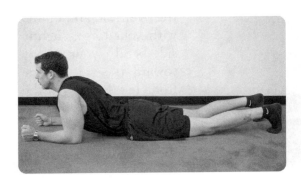
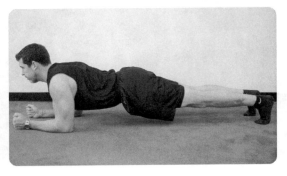

3D HIP FLEXOR STRETCH

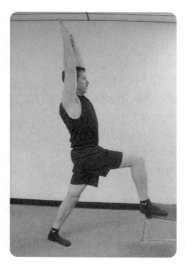

Begin with one foot on a chair with the knee bent. The other foot is behind you, with the foot slightly toed in and the back leg straight. Tighten your abdominals, and slightly tilt your pelvis backward. Once you have done this, move your pelvis slightly toward the front foot. You should feel a slight stretch in the groin of your back leg. From this position, there will be three separate movements of the upper body and arms. Keep your abdominals tight the entire time.

1. Hold both arms straight out in front of your chest. From here, raise both arms straight overhead together, then bring them back to the starting position and repeat.

2. Hold both arms straight out in front of your chest. Turn your arms and upper body away from your back leg. Turn your head so that it follows the same motions as your arms and torso. Return to the start and repeat.

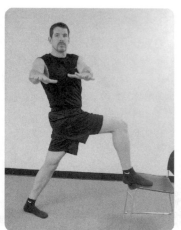

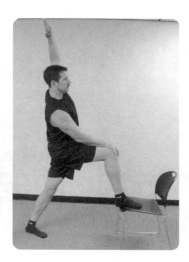

3. Hold the arm on the same side as the back leg straight up in the air. Place the other hand on the front knee. Keeping the overhead arm in line with your torso, slightly side-bend your body toward the side of the front leg. Return to the start and repeat.

Recommended Sets and Repetitions
1 set of 10 repetitions

Modification
In movement 2, you can keep your head and eyes still so that they aren't moving with your arms and torso. This will assist with balance.

Purpose
To elongate the hip flexor muscles by moving the upper attachment of the muscle away from the lower attachment, using the arms and the trunk. You should feel a stretch in the thigh and the groin of the back leg, as well as higher and deeper, possibly under the ribs.

DOWNWARD DOG

Start on your hands and knees with your hands directly under your shoulders and your knees directly under your hips. Your body should be square, like a box. Your weight should be evenly distributed between all four points of contact. Curl your toes under and raise your body up so that you are now on your hands and feet. Make sure your hands don't move back toward the feet. Push your hips up and back, trying to "pike" your body like a diver. Once you get your hips in the right position, tighten the quadriceps as you gently lower your heels to the floor. Don't lower your heels to the floor if it causes you to round your back. Check to make sure your feet are parallel and hip-width apart.

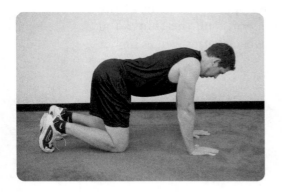

Recommended Duration
1 minute

Modification
None at this level

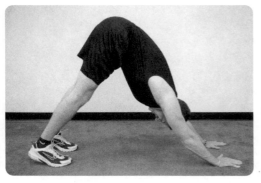

Purpose
To lengthen the muscles of the posterior aspect of the legs, while working the muscles of the upper body to create the stretch. You should feel the stretch in your calves and hamstrings. You should also feel that your upper body is continually working to maintain the proper position.

W9-BOL-813

Civil Disobedience
Solitude and Life without Principle

CIVIL DISOBEDIENCE
SOLITUDE AND LIFE WITHOUT PRINCIPLE

HENRY DAVID THOREAU

LITERARY CLASSICS

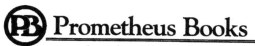

Prometheus Books
59 John Glenn Drive
Amherst, New York 14228-2197

Published 1998 by Prometheus Books

59 John Glenn Drive, Amherst, New York 14228-2197,
716-691-0133. FAX: 716-691-0137

Library of Congress Cataloging-in Publication Data

Thoreau, Henry David, 1817–1862.
    [Writings of Henry David Thoreau]
    Civil disobedience, solitude, and life without principle / Henry David
Thoreau.
        p.   cm. — (Literary classics)
    Originally published: The writings of Henry David Thoreau. Boston :
Houghton Mifflin, 1906.
    Contents: Civil disobedience — Solitude — Life without principle.
    ISBN 1–57392–202–1 (acid-free paper)
    1. Civil disobedience. 2. Solitude. I. Title. II. Series: Literary classics
(Amherst, N.Y.)
PS3042   1998
818'.309—dc21   98–14423
                                                        CIP

Printed in the United States of America on acid-free paper

Prometheus's Literary Classics Series

HENRY DAVID THOREAU was born in Concord, Massachusetts, on July 12, 1817. Although he lived elsewhere for a short period of time, for most of his life he resided in Concord and neighboring towns. Thoreau's college years were spent at Harvard, where he met Ralph Waldo Emerson, head of the philosophical movement known as Transcendentalism. This philosophy, which claimed that ultimate reality is unknowable, advocated the primacy of the spiritual over the material and empirical. Thoreau lived with Emerson for a number of years and helped him to publish *The Dial*, a transcendental periodical to which Thoreau also contributed poems and essays.

Thoreau taught school briefly, and tutored, and even worked in his father's pencil factory, but writing was the way he wished to make his living. His famous residence at Walden Pond was undertaken in part to explore whether a life devoted primarily to writing was possible. From July 4, 1845, to September 6, 1847, Thoreau lived in a small cabin he had built on land Emerson owned near Walden Pond. The choice to live in seclusion added to Thoreau's reputation as an eccentric; but also added impetus for his writing.

Another event enhanced both these aspects of Thoreau's life: While living at Walden, he refused to pay a poll tax in protest of a government that allowed slavery and an imperialistic war such as that against Mexico, resulting in a one-night stay in the local jail. In the morning, over Thoreau's objections, his aunt paid the tax and he was released. "Resistance to Civil Government," later known as "Civil Disobedience," grew out of the experience. In this essay Thoreau emphasized personal ethics and responsibility, as well as the violation of unjust civil laws in order to effect their repeal. These novel ideas later influenced twentieth-century leaders Mahatma Gandhi and Martin Luther King Jr.

Thoreau's social protest and defiance of social mores continued throughout his life, as his ardent abolitionism evidences. In addition to participating in the Underground Railroad, Thoreau publicly supported John Brown's raid on Harper's Ferry with his "Plea for Captain John Brown" (1859). Thoreau died of tuberculosis at Concord on May 6, 1862.

Although he had devoted his life to writing, Thoreau was never able to make a living by it. His first book, *A Week on the Concord and Merrimack Rivers* (1849), was printed locally at his own expense, and only 219 of the 1,000 copies printed were sold. Even *Walden* (1854), although it received good reviews, sold very slowly. Most of Thoreau's other major works, *Excursions* (1863), *The Maine Woods* (1864), *Cape Cod* (1865), and *A Yankee in Canada* (1866) were published posthumously.

CONTENTS

CIVIL DISOBEDIENCE

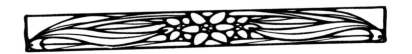

I HEARTILY ACCEPT THE MOTTO,—"That government is best which governs least;" and I should like to see it acted up to more rapidly and systematically. Carried out, it finally amounts to this, which also I believe,— "That government is best which governs not at all;" and when men are prepared for it, that will be the kind of government which they will have. Government is at best but an expedient; but most governments are usually, and all governments are sometimes, inexpedient. The objections which have been brought against a standing army, and they are many and weighty, and deserve to prevail, may also at last be brought against a standing government. The standing army is only an arm of the standing government. The government itself, which is only the mode which the people have chosen to execute their will, is equally liable to be abused and perverted before the people can act through it. Witness the present Mexican war, the work of comparatively a few individuals using the standing government as their tool; for, in the outset, the people would not have consented to this measure.

This American government,—what is it but a tradition, though a recent one, endeavoring to transmit itself unimpaired to posterity, but each instant losing some of its integrity? It has not the vitality and force of a single living man; for a single man can bend it to his will. It is a sort of wooden gun to the people themselves. But it is not the less necessary for this; for the people must have some complicated machinery or other, and hear its din, to satisfy that idea of government which they have. Governments show thus how successfully men can be imposed on, even impose on themselves, for their own advantage. It is excellent, we must all allow. Yet this government never of itself furthered any enterprise, but by the alacrity with which it got out of its way. *It* does not keep the country free. *It* does not settle the West. *It* does not educate. The character inherent in the American people has done all that has been accomplished; and it would have done somewhat more, if the government had not sometimes got in its way. For government is an expedient by which men would fain succeed in letting one another alone; and, as has been said, when it is most expedient, the governed are most let alone by it. Trade and commerce, if they were not made of India-rubber, would never manage to bounce over the obstacles which legislators are continually putting in their way; and, if one were to judge these men wholly by the effects of their actions and not partly by their intentions, they would deserve to be classed and punished with those mischievous persons who put obstructions on the railroads.

But, to speak practically and as a citizen, unlike those who call themselves no-government men, I ask for, not at once no government, but *at once* a better government. Let every man make known what kind of government would command his respect, and that will be one step toward obtaining it.

After all, the practical reason why, when the power is once in the hands of the people, a majority are permitted, and for a long period continue, to rule is not because they are most likely to be in the right, nor because this seems fairest to the minority, but because they are physically the strongest. But a government in which the majority rule in all cases cannot be based on justice, even as far as men understand it. Can there not be a government in which majorities do not virtually decide right and wrong, but conscience?—in which majorities decide only those questions to which the rule of expediency is applicable? Must the citizen ever for a moment, or in the least degree, resign his conscience to the legislator? Why has every man a conscience, then? I think that we should be men first, and subjects afterward. It is not desirable to cultivate a respect for the law, so much as for the right. The only obligation which I have a right to assume is to do at any time what I think right. It is truly enough said, that a corporation has no conscience; but a corporation of conscientious men is a corporation *with* a conscience. Law never made men a whit more just; and, by means of their respect for it, even the well-disposed are daily made the agents of injustice. A common and natural result of an undue respect for law is, that you may see a file of soldiers, colonel, captain, corporal, privates, powder-monkeys, and all, marching in admirable order over hill and dale to the wars, against their wills, ay, against their common sense and consciences, which makes it very steep marching indeed, and produces a palpitation of the heart. They have no doubt that it is a damnable business in which they are concerned; they are all peaceably inclined. Now, what are they? Men at all? or small movable forts and magazines, at the service of some unscrupulous man in power? Visit the Navy-Yard, and behold a marine, such a man as an American government can make, or such as it can make a man with its black arts,—a mere shadow and reminiscence of humanity, a man laid out alive and standing, and already, as one may say, buried under arms with funeral accompaniments, though it may be,—

"Not a drum was heard, not a funeral note,
    As his corse to the rampart we hurried;
Not a soldier discharged his farewell shot
    O'er the grave where our hero we buried."

The mass of men serve the state thus, not as men mainly, but as machines, with their bodies. They are the standing army, and the militia, jailors, constables, posse comitatus, etc. In most cases there is no free exercise whatever of the judgment or of the moral sense; but they put themselves on a level with wood and earth and stones; and wooden men can perhaps be manufactured that will serve the purpose as well. Such command no more respect than men of straw or a lump of dirt. They have the same sort of worth only as horses and dogs. Yet such as these even are commonly esteemed good citizens. Others—as most legislators, politicians, lawyers, ministers, and office-holders—serve the state chiefly with their heads; and, as they rarely make any moral distinctions, they are as likely to serve the Devil, without *intending* it, as God. A very few, as heroes, patriots, martyrs, reformers in the great sense, and *men*, serve the state with their consciences also, and so necessarily resist it for the most part; and they are commonly treated as enemies by it. A wise man will only be useful as a man, and will not submit to be "clay," and "stop a hole to keep the wind away," but leave that office to his dust at least:—

> "I am too high-born to be propertied,
> To be a secondary at control,
> Or useful serving-man and instrument
> To any sovereign state throughout the world."

He who gives himself entirely to his fellow-men appears to them useless and selfish; but he who gives himself partially to them is pronounced a benefactor and philanthropist.

How does it become a man to behave toward this

American government to-day? I answer, that he cannot without disgrace be associated with it. I cannot for an instant recognize that political organization as *my* government which is the *slave's* government also.

All men recognize the right of revolution; that is, the right to refuse allegiance to, and to resist, the government, when its tyranny or its inefficiency are great and unendurable. But almost all say that such is not the case now. But such was the case, they think, in the Revolution of '75. If one were to tell me that this was a bad government because it taxed certain foreign commodities brought to its ports, it is most probable that I should not make an ado about it, for I can do without them. All machines have their friction; and possibly this does enough good to counterbalance the evil. At any rate, it is a great evil to make a stir about it. But when the friction comes to have its machine, and oppression and robbery are organized, I say, let us not have such a machine any longer. In other words, when a sixth of the population of a nation which has undertaken to be the refuge of liberty are slaves, and a whole country is unjustly overrun and conquered by a foreign army, and subjected to military law, I think that it is not too soon for honest men to rebel and revolutionize. What makes this duty the more urgent is the fact that the country so overrun is not our own, but ours is the invading army.

Paley, a common authority with many on moral questions, in his chapter on the "Duty of Submission to Civil Government," resolves all civil obligation into expediency; and he proceeds to say, "that so long as the interest of the whole society requires it, that is, so long as the established government cannot be resisted or changed without public inconveniency, it is the will of God that the established government be obeyed, and no longer. . . . This principle being admitted, the justice of every particular case of resistance is reduced to a computation of the quantity of the danger and grievance on the one side, and of the probability and expense of redressing it on the other." Of this, he says, every man shall judge for himself. But Paley appears never to have contemplated those cases to which the rule of expediency does not apply, in which a people, as well as an individual, must do justice, cost what it may. If I have unjustly wrested a plank from a drowning man, I must restore it to him though I drown myself. This, according to Paley, would be inconvenient. But he that would save his life, in such a case, shall lose it. This people must cease to hold slaves, and to make war on Mexico, though it cost them their existence as a people.

In their practice, nations agree with Paley; but does anyone think that Massachusetts does exactly what is right at the present crisis?

> "A drab of state, a cloth-o'-silver slut,
> To have her train borne up, and her soul trail
>   in the dirt."

Practically speaking, the opponents to a reform in Massachusetts are not a hundred thousand politicians at the South, but a hundred thousand merchants and farmers here, who are more interested in commerce and agriculture than they are in humanity, and are not prepared to do justice to the slave and to Mexico, *cost what it may.* I quarrel not with far-off foes, but with those who, near at home, cooperate with, and do the bidding of, those far away, and without whom the latter would be harmless. We are accustomed to say, that the mass of men are unprepared; but improvement is slow, because the few are not materially wiser or better than the many. It is not so important that many should be as good as you, as that there be some absolute goodness somewhere; for that will leaven the whole lump. There are thousands who are *in opinion* opposed to slavery and to the war, who yet in effect do nothing to put an end to them; who, esteeming themselves children of Washington and Franklin, sit down with their hands in their pockets, and say that they know not what to do, and do nothing; who even postpone the question of freedom to the question of free-trade, and quietly read the prices-current along with the latest advices from Mexico, after dinner, and, it may be, fall asleep over them both. What is the price-current of an honest man and patriot to-day? They hesitate, and they regret, and sometimes they petition; but they do nothing in earnest and with effect. They will wait, well disposed, for others to remedy the evil, that they may no longer have it to regret. At most, they give only a cheap vote, and a feeble countenance and God-speed, to the right, as it goes by them. There are nine hundred and ninety-nine patrons of virtue to one virtuous man. But it is easier to deal with the real possessor of a thing than with the temporary guardian of it.

All voting is a sort of gaming, like checkers or back-gammon, with a slight moral tinge to it, a playing with right and wrong, with moral questions; and betting naturally accompanies it. The character of the voters is not staked. I cast my vote, perchance, as I think right; but I am not vitally concerned that that right should prevail. I am willing to leave it to the majority. Its obligation, therefore, never exceeds that of expediency. Even voting *for the right* is *doing* nothing for it. It is only expressing to men feebly your desire that it should prevail. A wise man will not leave the right to the mercy of chance, nor wish it to prevail through the power of the majority. There is but little virtue in the action of masses of men. When the majority shall at length vote for the abolition of slavery, it will be because they are indifferent to slavery, or because there is but little slavery left to be abolished by their vote. *They* will then be the only slaves. Only *his* vote can hasten the abolition of slavery who asserts his own freedom by his vote.

I hear of a convention to be held at Baltimore, or elsewhere, for the selection of a candidate for the Presidency, made up chiefly of editors, and men who are politicians by profession; but I think, what is it to any independent, intelligent, and respectable man what decision they may come to? Shall we not have the advantage of his wisdom and honesty, nevertheless? Can we not count upon some independent votes? Are there not many individuals in the country who do not attend conventions? But no: I find that the respectable man, so called, has immediately drifted from his position, and despairs of his country, when his country has more reason to despair of him. He forthwith adopts one of the candidates thus selected as the only *available* one, thus proving that he is himself *available* for any purposes of the demagogue. His vote is of no more worth than that of any unprincipled foreigner or hireling native, who may have been bought. O for a man who is a *man*, and, as my neighbor says, has a bone in his back which you cannot pass your hand through! Our statistics are at fault: the population has been returned too large. How many *men* are there to a square thousand miles in this country? Hardly one. Does not America offer any inducement for men to settle here? The American has dwindled into an Odd Fellow,—one who may be known by the development of his organ of gregariousness, and a manifest lack of intellect and cheerful self-reliance; whose first and chief concern, on coming into the world, is to see that the Almshouses are in good repair; and, before yet he has lawfully donned the virile garb, to collect a fund for the support of the widows and orphans that may be; who, in short, ventures to live only by the aid of the Mutual Insurance company, which has promised to bury him decently.

It is not a man's duty, as a matter of course, to devote himself to the eradication of any, even the most enormous wrong; he may still properly have other concerns to engage him; but it is his duty, at least, to wash his hands of it, and, if he gives it no thought longer, not to give it practically his support. If I devote myself to other pursuits and contemplations, I must first see, at least, that

I do not pursue them sitting upon another man's shoulders. I must get off him first, that he may pursue his contemplations too. See what gross inconsistency is tolerated. I have heard some of my townsmen say, "I should like to have them order me out to help put down an insurrection of the slaves, or to march to Mexico;—see if I would go;" and yet these very men have each, directly by their allegiance, and so indirectly, at least, by their money, furnished a substitute. The soldier is applauded who refuses to serve in an unjust war by those who do not refuse to sustain the unjust government which makes the war; is applauded by those whose own act and authority he disregards and sets at naught; as if the state were penitent to that degree that it hired one to scourge it while it sinned, but not to that degree that it left off sinning for a moment. Thus, under the name of Order and Civil Government, we are all made at last to pay homage to and support our own meanness. After the first blush of sin comes its indifference; and from immoral it becomes, as it were, *un*moral, and not quite unnecessary to that life which we have made.

The broadest and most prevalent error requires the most disinterested virtue to sustain it. The slight reproach to which the virtue of patriotism is commonly liable, the noble are most likely to incur. Those who, while they disapprove of the character and measures of a government, yield to it their allegiance and support are undoubtedly its most conscientious supporters, and so frequently the most serious obstacles to reform. Some are petitioning the state to dissolve the Union, to disregard the requisitions of the President. Why do they not dissolve it themselves,—the union between themselves and the state,—and refuse to pay their quota into its treasury? Do not they stand in the same relation to the state that the state does to the Union? And have not the same reasons prevented the state from resisting the Union which have prevented them from resisting the state?

How can a man be satisfied to entertain an opinion merely, and enjoy *it*? Is there any enjoyment in it, if his opinion is that he is aggrieved? If you are cheated out of a single dollar by your neighbor, you do not rest satisfied with knowing that you are cheated, or with saying that you are cheated, or even with petitioning him to pay you your due; but you take effectual steps at once to obtain the full amount, and see that you are never cheated again. Action from principle, the perception and the performance of right, changes things and relations; it is essentially revolutionary, and does not consist wholly with anything which was. It not only divides states and churches, it divides families; ay, it divides the *individual*, separating the diabolical in him from the divine.

Unjust laws exist: shall we be content to obey them, or shall we endeavor to amend them, and obey them until we have succeeded, or shall we transgress them at once? Men generally, under such a government as this, think that they ought to wait until they have persuaded the majority to alter them. They think that, if they should resist, the remedy would be worse than the evil. But it is the fault of the government itself that the remedy *is* worse than the evil. *It* makes it worse. Why is it not more apt to anticipate and provide for reform? Why does it not cherish its wise minority? Why does it cry and resist before it is hurt? Why does it not encourage its citizens to be on the alert to point out its faults, and *do* better than it would have them? Why does it always crucify Christ, and excommunicate Copernicus and Luther, and pronounce Washington and Franklin rebels?

One would think, that a deliberate and practical denial of its authority was the only offense never contemplated by government; else, why has it not assigned its definite, its suitable and proportionate penalty? If a man who has no property refuses but once to earn nine shillings for the state, he is put in prison for a period unlimited by any law that I know, and determined only by the discretion of those who placed him there; but if he should steal ninety times nine shillings from the state, he is soon permitted to go at large again.

If the injustice is part of the necessary friction of the machine of government, let it go, let it go: perchance it will wear smooth,—certainly the machine will wear out. If the injustice has a spring, or a pulley, or a rope, or a crank, exclusively for itself, then perhaps you may consider whether the remedy will not be worse than the evil; but if it is of such a nature that it requires you to be the agent of injustice to another, then, I say, break the law. Let your life be a counter friction to stop the machine. What I have to do is to see, at any rate, that I do not lend myself to the wrong which I condemn.

As for adopting the ways which the state has provided for remedying the evil, I know not of such ways.

They take too much time, and a man's life will be gone. I have other affairs to attend to. I came into this world, not chiefly to make this a good place to live in, but to live in it, be it good or bad. A man has not everything to do, but something; and because he cannot do *every-thing*, it is not necessary that he should do *something* wrong. It is not my business to be petitioning the Governor or the Legislature any more than it is theirs to petition me; and if they should not hear my petition, what should I do then? But in this case the state has provided no way: its very Constitution is the evil. This may seem to be harsh and stubborn and unconciliatory; but it is to treat with the utmost kindness and consideration the only spirit that can appreciate or deserves it. So is all change for the better, like birth and death, which convulse the body.

I do not hesitate to say, that those who call themselves Abolitionists should at once effectually withdraw their support, both in person and property, from the government of Massachusetts and not wait till they constitute a majority of one, before they suffer the right to prevail through them. I think that it is enough if they have God on their side, without waiting for that other one. Moreover, any man more right than his neighbors constitutes a majority of one already.

I meet this American government, or its representative, the state government, directly, and face to face, once a year—no more—in the person of its tax-gatherer; this is the only mode in which a man situated as I am necessarily meets it; and it then says distinctly, Recognize me; and the simplest, most effectual, and, in the present posture of affairs, the indispensablest mode of treating with it on this head, of expressing your little satisfaction with and love for it, is to deny it then. My civil neighbor, the tax-gatherer, is the very man I have to deal with,—for it is, after all, with men and not with parchment that I quarrel,—and he has voluntarily chosen to be an agent of the government. How shall he ever know well what he is and does as an officer of the government, or as a man, until he is obliged to consider whether he shall treat me, his neighbor, for whom he has respect, as a neighbor and well-disposed man, or as a maniac and disturber of the peace, and see if he can get over this obstruction to his neighborliness without a ruder and more impetuous thought or speech corresponding with his action. I know this well, that if one thousand, if one hundred, if ten men whom I could name,—if ten *honest* men only,—ay, if *one* HONEST man, in this State of Massachusetts, *ceasing to hold slaves,* were actually to withdraw from this copartnership, and be locked up in the county jail therefor, it would be the abolition of slavery in America. For it matters not how small the beginning may seem to be: what is once well done is done forever. But we love better to talk about it: that we say is our mission. Reform keeps many scores of newspapers in its service, but not one man. If my esteemed neighbor, the State's ambassador, who will devote his days to the settlement of the question of human rights in the Council Chamber, instead of being threatened with the prisons of Carolina, were to sit down the prisoner of Massachusetts, that State which is so anxious to foist the sin of slavery upon her sister,—though at present she can discover only an act of inhospitality to be the ground of a quarrel with her,—the Legislature would not wholly waive the subject the following winter.

Under a government which imprisons any unjustly, the true place for a just man is also a prison. The proper place to-day, the only place which Massachusetts has provided for her freer and less desponding spirits, is in her prisons, to be put out and locked out of the State by her own act, as they have already put themselves out by their principles. It is there that the fugitive slave, and the Mexican prisoner on parole, and the Indian come to plead the wrongs of his race should find them; on that separate, but more free and honorable ground, where the State places those who are not *with* her, but *against* her,—the only house in a slave State in which a free man can abide with honor. If any think that their influence would be lost there, and their voices no longer afflict the ear of the State, that they would not be as an enemy within its walls, they do not know by how much truth is stronger than error, nor how much more eloquently and effectively he can combat injustice who has experienced a little in his own person. Cast your whole vote, not a strip of paper merely, but your whole influence. A minority is powerless while it conforms to the majority; it is not even a minority then; but it is irresistible when it clogs by its whole weight. If the alternative is to keep all just men in prison, or give up war and slavery, the State will not hesitate which to choose. If a thousand men were not to pay their tax-bills this year, that would not be a violent and bloody measure, as it would be to pay them, and enable the State to commit violence and shed innocent blood. This is, in fact, the definition of a peaceable revolution, if any such is possible. If the tax-gatherer, or any other public officer, asks me, as one has done, "But what shall I do?" my answer is, "If you really wish to do anything, resign your office." When the subject has refused allegiance, and the officer has resigned his office, then the revolution is accomplished. But even suppose blood should flow. Is there not a sort of blood shed when the conscience is wounded? Through this wound a man's real manhood and immortality flow out, and he bleeds to an everlasting death. I see this blood flowing now.

I have contemplated the imprisonment of the offender, rather than the seizure of his goods,—though both will serve the same purpose,—because they who assert the purest right, and consequently are most dangerous to a corrupt State, commonly have not spent much time in accumulating property. To such the State renders comparatively small service, and a slight tax is wont to appear exorbitant, particularly if they are obliged to earn it by special labor with their hands. If there were one who lived wholly without the use of money, the State itself would hesitate to demand it of him. But the rich man—not to make any invidious comparison—is always sold to the institution which makes him rich. Absolutely speaking, the more money, the less virtue; for money comes between a man and his objects, and obtains them for him; and it was certainly no great virtue to obtain it. It puts to rest many questions which he would otherwise be taxed to answer; while the only new question which it puts is the hard but superfluous one, how to spend it. Thus his moral ground is taken from under his feet. The opportunities of living are diminished in proportion as what are called the "means" are increased. The best thing a man can do for his culture when he is rich is to endeavor to carry out those schemes which he entertained when he was poor. Christ answered the Herodians according to their condition. "Show me the tribute-money," said he;—and one took a penny out of his pocket;—if you use money which has the image of Caesar on it and which he has made current and valuable, that is, *if you are men of the State,* and gladly enjoy the advantages of Caesar's government, then pay him back some of his own when he demands it. "Render therefore to Caesar that which is Caesar's, and to God those things which are God's,"— leaving them no wiser than before as to which was which; for they did not wish to know.

When I converse with the freest of my neighbors, I perceive that, whatever they may say about the magnitude and seriousness of the question, and their regard for the public tranquillity, the long and the short of the matter is, that they cannot spare the protection of the existing government, and they dread the consequences to their property and families of disobedience to it. For my own part, I should not like to think that I ever rely on the protection of the State. But, if I deny the authority of the State when it presents its tax-bill, it will soon take and waste all my property, and so harass me and my children without end. This is hard. This makes it impossible for a man to live honestly, and at the same time comfortably, in outward respects. It will not be worth the while to accumulate property; that would be sure to go again. You must hire or squat somewhere, and raise but a small crop, and eat that soon. You must live within yourself, and depend upon yourself always tucked up and ready for a start, and not have many affairs. A man may grow rich in Turkey even, if he will be in all respects a good subject of the Turkish government. Confucius said: "If a state is governed by the principles of reason, poverty and misery are subjects of shame; if a state is not governed by the principles of reason, riches and honors are the subjects of shame." No: until I want the protection of Massachusetts to be extended to me in some distant Southern port, where my liberty is endangered, or until I am bent solely on building up an estate at home by peaceful enterprise, I can afford to refuse allegiance to Massachusetts, and her right to my property and life. It costs me less in every sense to incur the penalty of disobedience to the State than it would to obey. I should feel as if I were worth less in that case.

Some years ago, the State met me in behalf of the Church, and commanded me to pay a certain sum toward the support of a clergyman whose preaching my father attended, but never I myself. "Pay," it said, "or be locked up in the jail." I declined to pay, But, unfortunately, another man saw fit to pay it. I did not see why the schoolmaster should be taxed to support the priest, and not the priest the schoolmaster; for I was not the State's schoolmaster, but I supported myself by voluntary subscription. I did not see why the lyceum should not present its tax-bill, and have the State to back its demand, as well as the Church. However, at the request of the selectmen, I condescended to make some such statement as this in writing:—"Know all men by these presents, that I, Henry Thoreau, do not wish to be regarded as a member of any incorporated society which I have not joined." This I gave to the town clerk; and he has it. The State, having thus learned that I did not wish to be regarded as a member of that church, has never made a like demand on me since; though it said that it must adhere to its original presumption that time. If I had known how to name them, I should have signed off in detail from all the societies which I never signed on to; but I did not know where to find a complete list.

I have paid no poll-tax for six years. I was put into a jail once on this account, for one night; and, as I stood considering the walls of solid stone, two or three feet thick, the door of wood and iron, a foot thick, and the iron grating which strained the light, I could not help being struck with the foolishness of that institution which treated me as if I were mere flesh and blood and bones, to be locked up. I wondered that it should have concluded at length that this was the best use it could put me to, and had never thought to avail itself of my services in some way. I saw that, if there was a wall of stone between me and my townsmen, there was a still more difficult one to climb or break through before they could get to be as free as I was. I did not for a moment feel confined, and the walls seemed a great waste of stone and mortar. I felt as if I alone of all my townsmen had paid my tax. They plainly did not know how to treat me, but behaved like persons who are underbred. In every threat and in every compliment there was a blunder; for they thought that my chief desire was to stand the other side of that stone wall. I could not but smile to see how industriously they locked the door on my meditations, which followed them out again without let or hindrance, and *they* were really all that was dangerous. As they could not reach me, they had resolved to punish my body; just as boys, if they cannot come at some person against whom they have a spite, will abuse his dog. I saw that the State was half-witted, that it was timid as a lone woman with her silver spoons, and that it did not know its friends from its foes, and I lost all my remaining respect for it, and pitied it.

Thus the State never intentionally confronts a man's sense, intellectual or moral, but only his body, his senses. It is not armed with superior wit or honesty, but with superior physical strength. I was not born to be forced. I will breathe after my own fashion. Let us see who is the strongest. What force has a multitude? They only can force me who obey a higher law than I. They force me to become like themselves. I do not hear of *men* being *forced* to live this way or that by masses of men. What sort of life were that to live? When I meet a government which says to me, "Your money or your life," why should I be in haste to give it my money? It may be in a great strait, and not know what to do: I cannot help that. It must help itself; do as I do. It is not worth the while to snivel about it. I am not responsible for the successful working of the machinery of society. I am not the son of the engineer. I perceive that, when an acorn and a chestnut fall side by side, the one does not remain inert to make way for the other, but both obey their own laws, and spring and grow and flourish as best they can, till one, perchance, overshadows and destroys the other. If a plant cannot live according to its nature, it dies; and so a man.

The night in prison was novel and interesting enough. The prisoners in their shirt-sleeves were enjoying a chat and the evening air in the doorway, when I entered. But the jailer said, "Come, boys, it is time to lock up;" and so they dispersed, and I heard the sound of their steps returning into the hollow apartments. My room-mate was introduced to me by the jailer as "a first-rate fellow and a clever man." When the door was locked, he showed me where to hang my hat, and how he managed matters there. The rooms were white-washed once a month; and this one, at least, was the whitest, most simply furnished, and probably the neatest apartment in the town. He naturally wanted to know where I came from, and what brought me there; and, when I had told him, I asked him in my turn how he came there, presuming him to be an honest man, of course; and, as the world goes, I believe he was. "Why," said he, "they accuse me of burning a barn; but I never did it." As near as I could discover, he had probably gone to bed in a barn when drunk, and smoked his pipe there; and so a barn was burnt. He had the reputation of being a clever man, had been there some three months waiting for his trial to come on, and would have to wait as much longer; but he was quite domesticated and contented, since he got his board for nothing, and thought that he was well treated.

He occupied one window, and I the other; and I saw that if one stayed there long, his principal business would be to look out the window. I had soon read all the tracts that were left there, and examined where former prisoners had broken out, and where a grate had been sawed off, and heard the history of the various occupants of that room; for I found that even here there was a history and a gossip which never circulated beyond the walls of the jail. Probably this is the only house in the town where verses are composed, which are afterward printed in a circular form, but not published. I was shown quite a long list of verses which were composed by some young men who had been detected in an attempt to escape, who avenged themselves by singing them.

I pumped my fellow-prisoner as dry as I could, for fear I should never see him again; but at length he showed me which was my bed, and left me to blow out the lamp.

It was like traveling into a far country, such as I had never expected to behold, to lie there for one night. It seemed to me that I never had heard the town-clock strike before, nor the evening sounds of the village; for we slept with the windows open, which were inside the grating. It was to see my native village in the light of the Middle Ages, and our Concord was turned into a Rhine stream, and visions of knights and castles passed before me. They were the voices of old burghers that I heard in the streets. I was an involuntary spectator and auditor of whatever was done and said in the kitchen of the adjacent village-inn,—a wholly new and rare experience to me. It was a closer view of my native town. I was fairly inside of it. I never had seen its institutions before. This is one of its peculiar institutions; for it is a shire town. I began to comprehend what its inhabitants were about.

In the morning, our breakfasts were put through the hole in the door, in small oblong-square tin pans, made to fit, and holding a pint of chocolate, with brown bread, and an iron spoon. When they called for the vessels again, I was green enough to return what bread I had left; but my comrade seized it, and said that I should lay that up for lunch or dinner. Soon after he was let out to work at haying in a neighboring field, whither he went every day, and would not be back till noon; so he bade me good-day, saying that he doubted if he should see me again.

When I came out of prison,—for some one interfered, and paid that tax,—I did not perceive that great changes had taken place on the common, such as he observed who went in a youth and emerged a tottering and gray-headed man; and yet a change had to my eyes

come over the scene,—the town, and State, and country,
—greater than any that mere time could effect. I saw yet
more distinctly the State in which I lived. I saw to what
extent the people among whom I lived could be trusted
as good neighbors and friends; that their friendship was
for summer weather only; that they did not greatly propose to do right; that they were a distinct race from me
by their prejudices and superstitions, as the Chinamen
and Malays are; that in their sacrifices to humanity they
ran no risks, not even to their property; that after all they
were not so noble but they treated the thief as he had
treated them, and hoped, by a certain outward obser-
vance and a few prayers, and by walking in a particular
straight though useless path from time to time, to save
their souls. This may be to judge my neighbors harshly;
for I believe that many of them are not aware that they
have such an institution as the jail in their village.

It was formerly the custom in our village, when a
poor debtor came out of jail, for his acquaintances to
salute him, looking through their fingers, which were
crossed to represent the grating of a jail window, "How
do ye do?" My neighbors did not thus salute me, but first
looked at me, and then at one another, as if I had returned from a long journey. I was put into jail as I was
going to the shoemaker's to get a shoe which was
mended. When I was let out the next morning, I pro-
ceeded to finish my errand, and, having put on my
mended shoe, joined a huckleberry party, who were im-
patient to put themselves under my conduct; and in half
an hour,—for the horse was soon tackled,—was in the

midst of a huckleberry field, on one of our highest hills, two miles off, and then the State was nowhere to be seen.

This is the whole history of "My Prisons."

I have never declined paying the highway tax, because I am as desirous of being a good neighbor as I am of being a bad subject; and as for supporting schools, I am doing my part to educate my fellow-countrymen now. It is for no particular item in the tax-bill that I refuse to pay it. I simply wish to refuse allegiance to the State, to withdraw and stand aloof from it effectually. I do not care to trace the course of my dollar, if I could, till it buys a man or a musket to shoot with,—the dollar is innocent,—but I am concerned to trace the effects of my allegiance. In fact, I quietly declare war with the State, after my fashion, though I will still make what use and get what advantage of her I can, as is usual in such cases.

If others pay the tax which is demanded of me, from a sympathy with the State, they do but what they have already done in their own case, or rather they abet injustice to a greater extent than the State requires. If they pay the tax from a mistaken interest in the individual taxed, to save his property, or prevent his going to jail, it is because they have not considered wisely how far they let their private feelings interfere with the public good.

This, then, is my position at present. But one cannot be too much on his guard in such a case, lest his action be biased by obstinacy or an undue regard for the opinions of men. Let him see that he does only what belongs to himself and to the hour.

I think sometimes, Why, this people mean well, they are only ignorant; they would do better if they knew how: why give your neighbors this pain to treat you as they are not inclined to? But I think again, This is no reason why I should do as they do, or permit others to suffer much greater pain of a different kind. Again, I sometimes say to myself, When many millions of men, without heat, without ill will, without personal feeling of any kind, demand of you a few shillings only, without the possibility, such is their constitution, of retracting or altering their present demand, and without the possibility, on your side, of appeal to any other millions, why expose yourself to this overwhelming brute force? You do not resist cold and hunger, the winds and the waves, thus obstinately; you quietly submit to a thousand similar necessities. You do not put your head into the fire. But just in proportion as I regard this as not wholly a brute force, but partly a human force, and consider that I have relations to those millions as to so many millions of men, and not of mere brute or inanimate things, I see that appeal is possible, first and instantaneously, from them to the Maker of them, and, secondly, from them to themselves. But if I put my head deliberately into the fire, there is no appeal to fire or to the Maker of fire, and I have only myself to blame. If I could convince myself that I have any right to be satisfied with men as they are, and to treat them accordingly, and not according, in some respects, to my requisitions and expectations of what they and I ought to be, then, like a good Mussulman and fatalist, I should endeavor to be satisfied with things as they are, and say it is the will of God. And, above all, there is this difference between resisting this and a purely brute or natural force, that I can resist this with some effect; but I cannot expect, like Orpheus, to change the nature of the rocks and trees and beasts.

I do not wish to quarrel with any man or nation. I do not wish to split hairs, to make fine distinctions, or set myself up as better than my neighbors. I seek rather, I may say, even an excuse for conforming to the laws of the land. I am but too ready to conform to them. Indeed, I have reason to suspect myself on this head; and each year, as the tax-gatherer comes round, I find myself disposed to review the acts and position of the general and State governments, and the spirit of the people, to discover a pretext for conformity.

> "We must affect our country as our parents,
> And if at any time we alienate
> Our love or industry from doing it honor,
> We must respect effects and teach the soul
> Matter of conscience and religion,
> And not desire of rule or benefit."

I believe that the State will soon be able to take all my work of this sort out of my hands, and then I shall be no better a patriot than my fellow-countrymen. Seen from a lower point of view, the Constitution, with all its faults, is very good; the law and the courts are very respectable; even this State and this American government are, in many respects, very admirable, and rare things, to be thankful for, such as a great many have described them; but seen from a point of view a little higher, they are what I have described them; seen from a higher still, and the highest, who shall say what they are, or that they are worth looking at or thinking of at all?

However, the government does not concern me much, and I shall bestow the fewest possible thoughts on it. It is not many moments that I live under a government, even in this world. If a man is thought-free, fancy-free, imagination-free, that which *is not* never for a long time appearing *to be* to him, unwise rulers or reformers cannot fatally interrupt him.

I know that most men think differently from myself; but those whose lives are by profession devoted to the study of these or kindred subjects content me as little as any. Statesmen and legislators, standing so completely within the institution, never distinctly and nakedly behold it. They speak of moving society, but have no resting-place without it. They may be men of a certain experience and discrimination, and have no doubt invented ingenious and even useful systems, for which we sincerely thank them; but all their wit and usefulness lie within certain not very wide limits. They are wont to forget that the world is not governed by policy and expediency. Webster never goes behind government, and so cannot speak with authority about it. His words are wisdom to those legislators who contemplate no essential reform in the existing government; but for thinkers, and those who legislate for all time, he never once glances at the subject. I know of those whose serene and wise speculations on this theme would soon reveal the limits of his mind's range and hospitality. Yet, compared with the cheap professions of most reformers, and the still cheaper wisdom and eloquence of politicians in general, his are almost the only sensible and valuable words, and we thank Heaven for him. Comparatively, he is always strong, original, and, above all, practical. Still, his quality is not wisdom, but prudence. The lawyer's truth is not Truth, but consistency or a consistent expediency. Truth is always in harmony with herself, and is not concerned chiefly to reveal the justice that may consist with wrong-doing. He well deserves to be called, as he has been called, the Defender of the Constitution. There are really no blows to be given by him but defensive ones. He is not a leader, but a follower. His leaders are the men of '87. "I have never made an effort," he says, "and never propose to make an effort; I have never countenanced an effort, and never mean to countenance an effort, to disturb the arrangement as originally made, by which the various States came into the Union." Still thinking of the sanction which the Constitution gives to slavery, he says, "Because it was a part of the original compact,—let it stand." Notwithstanding his special acuteness and ability, he is unable to take a fact out of its merely political relations, and behold it as it lies absolutely to be disposed of by the intellect,—what, for instance, it behooves a man to do here in America to-day with regard to slavery,—but ventures, or is driven, to make some such desperate answer as the following, while professing to speak absolutely, and as a private man,—from which what new and singular code of social duties might be inferred? "The manner," says he, "in which the governments of those States where slavery exists are to regulate it is for their own consideration, under their responsibility to their constituents, to the general laws of propriety, humanity, and justice, and to God. Associations formed elsewhere, springing from a feeling of humanity, or other cause, have nothing whatever to do with it. They have never received any encouragement from me, and they never will."

They who know of no purer sources of truth, who have traced up its stream no higher, stand, and wisely stand, by the Bible and the Constitution, and drink at it there with reverence and humility; but they who behold where it comes trickling into this lake or that pool, gird up their loins once more, and continue their pilgrimage toward its fountainhead.

No man with a genius for legislation has appeared in America. They are rare in the history of the world. There are orators, politicians, and eloquent men, by the thousand; but the speaker has not yet opened his mouth to speak who is capable of settling the much-vexed questions of the day. We love eloquence for its own sake, and not for any truth which it may utter, or any heroism it may inspire. Our legislators have not yet learned the comparative value of free-trade and of freedom, of union, and of rectitude, to a nation. They have no genius or talent for comparatively humble questions of taxation and finance, commerce and manufactures and agriculture. If we were left solely to the wordy wit of legislators in Congress for our guidance, uncorrected by the seasonable experience and the effectual complaints of the people, America would not long retain her rank among the nations. For eighteen hundred years, though perchance I have no right to say it, the New Testament has been written; yet where is the legislator who has wisdom and practical talent enough to avail himself of the light which it sheds on the science of legislation?

The authority of government, even such as I am willing to submit to,—for I will cheerfully obey those who know and can do better than I, and in many things even those who neither know nor can do so well,—is still an impure one: to be strictly just, it must have the sanction and consent of the governed. It can have no pure right over my person and property but what I concede to it. The progress from an absolute to a limited monarchy, from a limited monarchy to a democracy, is a progress toward a true respect for the individual. Even the Chinese philosopher was wise enough to regard the individual as the basis of the empire. Is a democracy, such as we know it, the last improvement possible in government? Is it not possible to take a step further towards recognizing and organizing the rights of man? There will never be a really free and enlightened State until the State comes to recognize the individual as a higher and independent power, from which all its own power and authority are derived, and treats him accordingly. I please myself with imagining a State at last which can afford to be just to all men, and to treat the individual with respect as a neighbor; which even would not think it inconsistent with its own repose if a few were to live aloof from it, not meddling with it, nor embraced by it, who fulfilled all the duties of neighbors and fellow-men. A State which bore this kind of fruit, and suffered it to drop off as fast as it ripened, would prepare the way for a still more perfect and glorious State, which also I have imagined, but not yet anywhere seen.

SOLITUDE

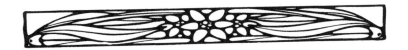

THIS IS A DELICIOUS EVENING, when the whole body is one sense, and imbibes delight through every pore. I go and come with a strange liberty in Nature, a part of herself. As I walk along the stony shore of the pond in my shirt-sleeves, though it is cool as well as cloudy and windy, and I see nothing special to attract me, all the elements are unusually congenial to me. The bullfrogs trump to usher in the night, and the note of the whip-poor-will is borne on the rippling wind from over the water. Sympathy with the fluttering alder and poplar leaves almost takes away my breath; yet, like the lake, my serenity is rippled but not ruffled. These small waves raised by the evening wind are as remote from storm as the smooth reflecting surface. Though it is now dark, the wind still blows and roars in the wood, the waves still dash, and some creatures lull the rest with their notes. The repose is never complete. The wildest animals do not repose, but seek their prey now; the fox, and skunk, and rabbit, now roam the fields and woods without fear. They are Nature's watchmen,—links which connect the days of animated life.

When I return to my house I find that visitors have been there and left their cards, either a bunch of flowers, or a wreath of evergreen, or a name in pencil on a yellow walnut leaf or a chip. They who come rarely to the woods take some little piece of the forest into their hands to play with by the way, which they leave, either intentionally or accidentally. One has peeled a willow wand, woven it into a ring, and dropped it on my table. I could always tell if visitors had called in my absence, either by the bended twigs or grass, or the print of their shoes, and generally of what sex or age or quality they were by some slight trace left, as a flower dropped, or a bunch of grass plucked and thrown away, even as far off as the railroad, half a mile distant, or by the lingering odor of a cigar or pipe. Nay, I was frequently notified of the passage of a traveller along the highway sixty rods off by the scent of his pipe.

There is a commonly sufficient space about us. Our horizon is never quite at our elbows. The thick wood is not just at our door, nor the pond, but somewhat is always clearing, familiar and worn by us, appropriated and fenced in some way, and reclaimed from Nature. For what reason have I this vast range and circuit, some square miles of unfrequented forest, for my privacy, abandoned to me by men? My nearest neighbor is a mile distant, and no house is visible from any place but the hill-tops within half a mile of my own. I have my horizon bounded by woods all to myself, a distant view of the railroad where it touches the pond on the one hand, and of the fence which skirts the woodland road on the other. But for the most part it is as solitary where I live as on the prairies. It is as much Asia or Africa as New England. I have, as it were, my own sun and moon and stars and a little world all to myself. At night there was never a traveller passed my house, or knocked at my door, more than if I were the first or last man; unless it were in the spring when at long intervals some came from the village to fish for pouts,—they plainly fished much more in the Walden Pond of their own natures, and baited their hooks with darkness,—but they soon retreated, usually with light baskets, and left "the world to darkness and to me," and the black kernel of the night was never profaned by any human neighborhood. I believe that men are generally still a little afraid of the dark, though the witches are all hung, and Christianity and candles have been introduced.

Yet I experienced sometimes that the most sweet and tender, the most innocent and encouraging society may be found in any natural object, even for the poor misanthrope and most melancholy man. There can be no very black melancholy to him who lives in the midst of nature and has his senses still. There was never yet such a storm but it was Aeolian music to a healthy and innocent ear. Nothing can rightly compel a simple and brave man to a vulgar sadness. While I enjoy the friendship of the seasons I trust that nothing can make life a burden to me. The gentle rain which waters my beans and keeps me in the house to-day is not drear and melancholy, but good for me too. Though it prevents my hoeing them, it is of far more worth than my hoeing. If it should continue so long as to cause the seeds to rot in the ground and destroy the potatoes in the low lands, it would still be good for the grass on the uplands, and, being good for the grass, it would be good for me. Sometimes, when I compare myself with other men, it seems as if I were more favored by the gods than they, beyond any deserts that I am conscious of; as if I had a warrant and surety at their hands which my fellows have not, and were especially guided and guarded. I do not flatter myself, but if it be possible they flatter me. I have never felt lonesome, or in the least oppressed by a sense of solitude, but once, and that was a few weeks after I came to the woods, when, for an hour, I doubted if the near neighborhood of man was not essential to a serene and healthy life. To be alone was something unpleasant. But I was at the same time conscious of a slight insanity in my mood, and seemed to foresee my recovery. In the midst of a gentle rain while these thoughts prevailed, I was suddenly sensible of such sweet and beneficent society in Nature, in the very pattering of the drops, and in every sound and sight around my house, an infinite and unaccountable friendliness all at once like an atmosphere sustaining me, as made the fancied advantages of human neighborhood insignificant, and I have never thought of them since. Every little pine needle expanded and swelled with sympathy and befriended me.

I was so distinctly made aware of the presence of something kindred to me, even in scenes which we are accustomed to call wild and dreary, and also that the
nearest of blood to me and humanest was not a person
nor a villager, that I thought no place could ever be
strange to me again.—

> "Mourning untimely consumes the sad;
> Few are their days in the land of the living,
> Beautiful daughter of Toscar."

Some of my pleasantest hours were during the long
rainstorms in the spring or fall, which confined me to
the house for the afternoon as well as the forenoon,
soothed by their ceaseless roar and pelting; when an
early twilight ushered in a long evening in which many
thoughts had time to take root and unfold themselves.
In those driving northeast rains which tried the village
houses so, when the maids stood ready with mop and
pail in front entries to keep the deluge out, I sat behind
my door in my little house, which was all entry, and
thoroughly enjoyed its protection. In one heavy
thunder-shower the lightning struck a large pitch pine
across the pond, making a very conspicuous and perfectly regular spiral groove from top to bottom, an inch
or more deep, and four or five inches wide, as you would
groove a walking stick. I passed it again the other day,
and was struck with awe on looking up and beholding
that mark, now more distinct than ever, where a terrific
and resistless bolt came down out of the harmless sky

eight years ago. Men frequently say to me, "I should think you would feel lonesome down there, and want to be nearer to folks, rainy and snowy days and nights especially." I am tempted to reply to such,—This whole earth which we inhabit is but a point in space. How far apart, think you, dwell the two most distant inhabitants of yonder star, the breadth of whose disk cannot be appreciated by our instruments? Why should I feel lonely? is not our planet in the Milky Way? This which you put seems to me not to be the most important question. What sort of space is that which separates a man from his fellows and makes him solitary? I have found that no exertion of the legs can bring two minds much nearer to one another. What do we want most to dwell near to? Not to many men surely, the depot, the post-office, the bar-room, the meeting-house, the school-house, the grocery, Beacon Hill, or the Five Points, where men most congregate, but to the perennial source of our life, whence in all our experience we have found that to issue, as the willow stands near the water and sends out its roots in that direction. This will vary with different natures, but this is the place where a wise man will dig his cellar. . . . I one evening overtook one of my townsmen, who has accumulated what is called "a handsome property,"—though I never got a *fair* view of it,—on the Walden road, driving a pair of cattle to market, who inquired of me how I could bring my mind to give up so many of the comforts of life. I answered that I was very sure I liked it passably well; I was not joking. And so I went home to my bed, and left him to pick his way through the darkness and the mud to Brighton,—or Bright-town,—which place he would reach some time in the morning.

Any prospect of awakening or coming to life to a dead man makes indifferent all times and places. The place where that may occur is always the same, and indescribably pleasant to all our senses. For the most part we allow only outlying and transient circumstances to make our occasions. They are, in fact, the cause of our distraction. Nearest to all things is that power which fashions their being. *Next* to us the grandest laws are continually being executed. *Next* to us is not the workman whom we have hired, with whom we love so well to talk, but the workman whose work we are.

"How vast and profound is the influence of the subtile powers of Heaven and of Earth!"

"We seek to perceive them, and we do not see them; we seek to hear them, and we do not hear them; identified with the substance of things, they cannot be separated from them."

"They cause that in all the universe men purify and sanctify their hearts, and clothe themselves in their holiday garments to offer sacrifices and oblations to their ancestors. It is an ocean of subtile intelligences. They are everywhere, above us, on our left, on our right; they environ us on all sides."

We are the subjects of an experiment which is not a little interesting to me. Can we not do without the society of our gossips a little while under these circumstances,—have our own thought to cheer us? Confucius says truly, "Virtue does not remain as an abandoned orphan; it must of necessity have neighbors."

With thinking we may be beside ourselves in a sane sense. By a conscious effort of the mind we can stand aloof from actions and their consequences; and all things, good and bad, go by us like a torrent. We are not wholly involved in Nature. I may be either the driftwood in the stream, or Indra in the sky looking down on it. I *may* be affected by a theatrical exhibition; on the other hand, I *may not* be affected by an actual event which appears to concern me much more. I only know myself as a human entity; the scene, so to speak, of thoughts and affections; and am sensible of a certain doubleness by which I can stand as remote from myself as from another. However intense my experience, I am conscious of the presence and criticism of a part of me, which, as it were, is not a part of me, but a spectator, sharing no experience, but taking note of it, and that is no more I than it is you. When the play, it may be the tragedy, of life is over, the spectator goes his way. It was a kind of fiction, a work of the imagination only, so far as he was concerned. This doubleness may easily make us poor neighbors and friends sometimes.

I find it wholesome to be alone the greater part of the time. To be in company, even with the best, is soon wearisome and dissipating. I love to be alone. I never found the companion that was so companionable as solitude. We are for the most part more lonely when we go abroad among men than when we stay in our chambers. A man thinking or working is always alone, let him be where he will. Solitude is not measured by the miles of space that intervene between a man and his fellows. The really diligent student in one of the crowded hives of Cambridge College is as solitary as a dervis in the desert. The farmer can work alone in the field or the woods all day, hoeing or chopping, and not feel lonesome, because he is employed; but when he comes home at night he cannot sit down in a room alone, at the mercy of his thoughts, but must be where he can "see the folks," and recreate, and, as he thinks, remunerate himself for his day's solitude; and hence he wonders how the student can sit alone in the house all night and most of the day without ennui and "the blues;" but he does not realize that the student, though in the house, is still at work in *his* field, and chopping in *his* woods, as the farmer in his, and in turn seeks the same recreation and society that the latter does, though it may be a more condensed form of it.

Society is commonly too cheap. We meet at very short intervals, not having had time to acquire any new value for each other. We meet at meals three times a day, and give each other a new taste of that old musty cheese that we are. We have had to agree on a certain set of rules, called etiquette and politeness, to make this frequent meeting tolerable and that we need not come to open war. We meet at the post-office, and at the sociable, and about the fireside every night; we live thick and are in each other's way, and stumble over one another, and I think that we thus lose some respect for one another. Certainly less frequency would suffice for all important and hearty communications. Consider the girls in a factory,—never alone, hardly in their dreams. It would be better if there were but one inhabitant to a square mile, as where I live. The value of a man is not in his skin, that we should touch him.

I have heard of a man lost in the woods and dying of famine and exhaustion at the foot of a tree, whose loneliness was relieved by the grotesque visions with which, owing to bodily weakness, his diseased imagination surrounded him and which he believed to be real. So also, owing to bodily and mental health and strength, we may be continually cheered by a like but more normal and natural society, and come to know that we are never alone.

I have a great deal of company in my house; especially in the morning, when nobody calls. Let me suggest a few comparisons, that some one may convey an idea of my situation. I am no more lonely than the loon in the pond that laughs so loud, or than Walden Pond itself. What company has that lonely lake, I pray? And yet it has not the blue devils, but the blue angels in it, in the azure tint of its water. The sun is alone, except in thick weather, when there sometimes appear to be two, but one is a mock sun. God is alone—but the devil, he is far from being alone; he sees a great deal of company; he is legion. I am no more lonely than a single mullein or dandelion in a pasture, or a bean leaf, or a sorrel, or a horse-fly, or a bumblebee. I am no more lonely than the Mill Brook, or a weathercock, or the north star, or the south wind, or an April shower, or a January thaw or the first spider in a new house.

I have occasional visits in the long winter evenings, when the snow falls fast and the wind howls in the wood, from an old settler and original proprietor, who is reported to have dug Walden Pond, and stoned it, and fringed it with pine woods; who tells me stories of old time and of new eternity; and between us we manage to pass a cheerful evening with social mirth and pleasant views of things, even without apples or cider,—a most wise and humorous friend whom I love much, who keeps himself more secret than ever did Goffe or Whalley; and though he is thought to be dead none can show where he is buried. An elderly dame, too, dwells in my neighborhood, invisible to most persons, in whose odorous herb garden I love to stroll sometimes, gathering simples and listening to her fables; for she has a genius of unequalled fertility, and her memory runs back farther than mythology, and she can tell me the original of every fable, and on what fact every one is founded, for the incidents occurred when she was young. A ruddy and lusty old dame, who delights in all weathers and seasons, and is likely to outlive all her children yet.

The indescribable innocence and beneficence of Nature,—of sun and wind and rain, of summer and winter,—such health, such cheer, they afford forever! and such sympathy have they ever with our race, that all Nature would be affected and the sun's brightness fade, and the winds would sigh humanely, and the clouds rain tears, and the woods shed their leaves and put on mourning in midsummer, if any man should ever for a just cause grieve. Shall I not have intelligence with the earth? Am I not partly leaves and vegetable mould myself?

What is the pill which will keep us well, serene, contented? Not my or thy great-grandfather's, but our great-grandmother Nature's universal, vegetable, botanic medicines, by which she has kept herself young always, outlived so many old Parrs in her day, and fed her health with their decaying fatness. For my panacea, instead of one of those quack vials of a mixture dipped from Acheron and the Dead Sea, which come out of those long shallow black-schooner looking wagons which we sometimes see made to carry bottles, let me have a draught of undiluted morning air. Morning air! If men will not drink of this at the fountain-head of the day, why, then, we must even bottle up some and sell it in the shops, for the benefit of those who have lost their subscription ticket to morning time in this world. But remember, it will keep quite till noonday even in the coolest cellar, but drive out the stopples long ere that and follow westward the steps of Aurora. I am no worshipper of Hygeia, who was the daughter of that old herb-doctor Aesculapius, and who is represented on monuments holding a serpent in one hand, and in the other a cup out of which the serpent sometimes drinks; but rather of Hebe, cup-bearer to Jupiter, who was the daughter of Juno and wild lettuce, and who had the power of restoring gods and men to the vigor of youth. She was probably the only thoroughly sound-conditioned, healthy and robust young lady that ever walked the globe, and whenever she came it was spring.

LIFE WITHOUT PRINCIPLE

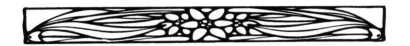

AT A LYCEUM, NOT LONG since, I felt that the lecturer had chosen a theme too foreign to himself, and so failed to interest me as much as he might have done. He described things not in or near to his heart, but toward his extremities and superficies. There was, in this sense, no truly central or centralizing thought in the lecture. I would have had him deal with his privatest experience, as the poet does. The greatest compliment that was ever paid me was when one asked me what *I thought,* and attended to my answer. I am surprised, as well as delighted, when this happens, it is such a rare use he would make of me, as if he were acquainted with the tool. Commonly, if men want anything of me, it is only to know how many acres I make of their land,—since I am a surveyor,—or, at most, what trivial news I have burdened myself with. They never will go to law for my meat; they prefer the shell. A man once came a considerable distance to ask me to lecture on Slavery; but on conversing with him, I found that he and his clique expected seven eighths of the lecture to be theirs, and only one eighth mine; so I declined. I take it for granted, when I am invited to lecture anywhere,— for I have had a little experience in that business,—that there is a desire to hear what *I think* on some subject, though I may be the greatest fool in the country,—and not that I should say pleasant things merely, or such as the audience will assent to; and I resolve, accordingly, that I will give them a strong dose of myself. They have sent for me, and engaged to pay for me, and I am determined that they shall have me, though I bore them beyond all precedent.

So now I would say something similar to you, my readers. Since *you* are my readers, and I have not been much of a traveler, I will not talk about people a thousand miles off, but come as near home as I can. As the time is short, I will leave out all the flattery, and retain all the criticism.

Let us consider the way in which we spend our lives.

This world is a place of business. What an infinite bustle! I am awaked almost every night by the panting of the locomotive. It interrupts my dreams. There is no sabbath. It would be glorious to see mankind at leisure for once. It is nothing but work, work, work. I cannot easily buy a blank-book to write thoughts in; they are commonly ruled for dollars and cents. An Irishman, seeing me making a minute in the fields, took it for granted that I was calculating my wages. If a man was tossed out of a window when an infant, and so made a cripple for life, or scared out of his wits by the Indians, it is regretted chiefly because he was thus incapacitated for—business! I think that there is nothing, not even crime, more opposed to poetry, to philosophy, ay, to life itself, than this incessant business.

There is a coarse and boisterous money-making fellow in the outskirts of our town, who is going to build a bank-wall under the hill along the edge of his meadow. The powers have put this into his head to keep him out of mischief, and he wishes me to spend three weeks digging there with him. The result will be that he will perhaps get some more money to hoard, and leave for his heirs to spend foolishly. If I do this, most will commend me as an industrious and hard-working man; but if I choose to devote myself to certain labors which yield more real profit, though but little money, they may be inclined to look on me as an idler. Nevertheless, as I do not need the police of meaningless labor to regulate me, and do not see anything absolutely praiseworthy in this fellow's undertaking any more than in many an enterprise of our own or foreign governments, however amusing it may be to him or them, I prefer to finish my education at a different school.

If a man walk in the woods for love of them half of each day, he is in danger of being regarded as a loafer; but if he spends his whole day as a speculator, shearing off those woods and making earth bald before her time, he is esteemed an industrious and enterprising citizen. As if a town had no interest in its forests but to cut them down!

Most men would feel insulted if it were proposed to employ them in throwing stones over a wall, and then in throwing them back, merely that they might earn their wages. But many are no more worthily employed now. For instance: just after sunrise, one summer morning, I noticed one of my neighbors walking beside his team, which was slowly drawing a heavy hewn stone swung under the axle, surrounded by an atmosphere of industry,—his day's work begun,—his brow commenced to sweat,—a reproach to all sluggards and idlers,—pausing abreast the shoulders of his oxen, and half turning round with a flourish of his merciful whip, while they gained their length on him. And I thought, Such is the labor which the American Congress exists to protect,—honest, manly toil,—honest as the day is long,—that makes his bread taste sweet, and keeps society sweet,—which all men respect and have consecrated; one of the sacred band, doing the needful but irksome drudgery. Indeed, I felt a slight reproach, because I observed this from a window, and was not abroad and stirring about a similar business. The day went by, and at evening I passed the yard of another neighbor, who keeps many servants, and spends much money foolishly, while he adds nothing to the common stock, and there I saw the stone of the morning lying beside a whimsical structure intended to adorn this Lord Timothy Dexter's premises, and the dignity forthwith departed from the teamster's labor, in my eyes. In my opinion, the sun was made to light worthier toil than this. I may add that his employer has since run off, in debt to a good part of town, and, after passing through Chancery, has settled somewhere else, there to become once more a patron of the arts.

The ways by which you may get money almost without exception lead downward. To have done anything by which you earned money *merely* is to have been truly idle or worse. If the laborer gets no more than the wages which his employer pays him, he is cheated, he cheats himself. If you would get money as a writer or lecturer, you must be popular, which is to go down perpendicularly. Those services which the community will most readily pay for, it is most disagreeable to render. You are paid for being something less than a man. The State does not commonly reward a genius any more wisely. Even the poet-laureate would rather not have to celebrate the accidents of royalty. He must be bribed with a pipe of wine; and perhaps another poet is called away from his muse to gauge that very pipe. As for my own business, even that kind of surveying which I could do with most satisfaction my employers do not want. They would prefer that I should do my work coarsely and not too well, ay, not well enough. When I observe that there are different ways of surveying, my employer commonly asks which will give him the most land, not which is most correct. I once invented a rule for measuring cord-wood, and tried to introduce it in Boston; but the measurer there told me that the sellers did not wish to have their wood measured correctly,— that he was already too accurate for them, and therefore they commonly got their wood measured in Charlestown before crossing the bridge.

The aim of the laborer should be, not to get his living, to get "a good job," but to perform well a certain work; and, even in a pecuniary sense, it would be economy for a town to pay its laborers so well that they would not feel that they were working for low ends, as for a livelihood merely, but for scientific, or even moral ends. Do not hire a man who does your work for money, but him who does it for love of it.

It is remarkable that there are few men so well employed, so much to their minds, but that a little money or fame would commonly buy them off from their present pursuit. I see advertisements for *active* young men, as if activity were the whole of a young man's capital. Yet I have been surprised when one has with confidence proposed to me, a grown man, to embark in some enterprise of his, as if I had absolutely nothing to do, my life having been a complete failure hitherto. What a doubtful compliment this to pay me! As if he had met me halfway across the ocean beating up against the wind, but bound nowhere, and proposed to me to go along with him! If I did, what do you think the underwriters would say? No, no! I am not without employment at this stage of the voyage. To tell the truth, I saw an advertisement for able-bodied seamen, when I was a boy, sauntering in my native port, and as soon as I came of age I embarked.

The community has no bribe that will tempt a wise man. You may raise money enough to tunnel a mountain, but you cannot raise money enough to hire a man who is minding *his own* business. An efficient and valuable man does what he can, whether the community pay him for it or not. The inefficient offer their inefficiency to the highest bidder, and are forever expecting to be put into office. One would suppose that they were rarely disappointed.

Perhaps I am more than usually jealous with respect to my freedom. I feel that my connection with and obligation to society are still very slight and transient. Those slight labors which afford me a livelihood, and by which it is allowed that I am to some extent serviceable to my contemporaries, are as yet commonly a pleasure to me, and I am not often reminded that they are a necessity. So far I am successful. But I foresee that if my wants should be much increased, the labor required to supply them would become a drudgery. If I should sell both my forenoons and afternoons to society, as most appear to do, I am sure that for me there would be nothing left worth living for. I trust that I shall never thus sell my birthright for a mess of pottage. I wish to suggest that a man may be very industrious, and yet not spend his time well. There is no more fatal blunderer than he who consumes the greater part of his life getting his living. All great enterprises are self-supporting. The poet, for instance, must sustain his body by his poetry, as a steam planing-mill feeds its boilers with the shavings it makes. You must get your living by loving. But as it is said of the merchants that ninety-seven in a hundred fail, so the life of men generally, tried by this standard, is a failure, and bankruptcy may be surely prophesied.

Merely to come into the world the heir of a fortune is not to be born, but to be still-born, rather. To be supported by the charity of friends, or a government-pension,—provided you continue to breathe,—by whatever fine synonyms you describe these relations, is to go into the almshouse. On Sundays the poor debtor goes to church to take an account of stock, and finds, of course, that his outgoes have been greater than his income. In the Catholic Church, especially, they go into Chancery, make a clean confession, give up all, and think to start again. Thus men will lie on their backs, talking about the fall of man, and never make an effort to get up.

As for the comparative demand which men make on life, it is an important difference between two, that the one is satisfied with a level success, that his marks can all be hit by point-blank shots, but the other, however low and unsuccessful his life may be, constantly elevates his aim, though at a very slight angle to the horizon. I should much rather be the last man,—though, as the Orientals say, "Greatness doth not approach him who is forever looking down; and all those who are looking high are growing poor."

It is remarkable that there is little or nothing to be remembered written on the subject of *getting* a living; how to make getting a living not merely honest and honorable, but altogether inviting and glorious; for if getting a living is not so, then living is not. One would think, from looking at literature, that this question had never disturbed a solitary individual's musings. Is it that men are too much disgusted with their experience to speak of it? The lesson of value which money teaches, which the Author of the Universe has taken so much pains to teach us, we are inclined to skip altogether. As for the means of living, it is wonderful how indifferent men of all classes are about it, even reformers, so called,—whether they inherit, or earn, or steal it. I think that Society has done nothing for us in this respect, or at least has undone what she has done. Cold and hunger seem more friendly to my nature than those methods which men have adopted and advise to ward them off.

The title *wise* is, for the most part, falsely applied. How can one be a wise man, if he does not know any better how to live than other men?—if he is only more cunning and intellectually subtle? Does Wisdom work in a treadmill? or does she teach how to succeed *by her example?* Is there any such thing as wisdom not applied to life? Is she merely the miller who grinds the finest logic? It is pertinent to ask if Plato got his *living* in a better way or more successfully than his contemporaries,—or did he succumb to the difficulties of life like other men? Did he seem to prevail over some of them merely by indifference, or by assuming grand airs? or find it easier to live, because his aunt remembered him in her will? The ways in which most men get their living, that is, live, are mere make-shifts, and a shirking of the real business of life,—chiefly because they do not know, but partly because they do not mean, any better.

The rush to California, for instance, and the attitude, not merely of merchants, but of philosophers and prophets, so called, in relation to it, reflect the greatest disgrace on mankind. That so many are ready to live by luck, and so get the means of commanding the labor of others less lucky, without contributing any value to society! And that is called enterprise! I know of no more startling development of the immortality of trade, and all the common modes of getting a living. The philosophy and poetry and religion of such a mankind are not worth the dust of a puff-ball. The hog that gets his living by rooting, stirring up the soil so, would be ashamed of such company. If I could command the wealth of all the worlds by lifting my finger, I would not pay *such* a price for it. Even Mahomet knew that God did not make this world in jest. It makes God to be a moneyed gentleman who scatters a handful of pennies in order to see mankind scramble for them. The world's raffle! A subsistence in the domains of Nature a thing to be raffled for! What a comment, what a satire, on our institutions! The conclusion will be, that mankind will hang itself upon a tree. And have all the precepts in all the Bibles taught men only this? and is the last and most admirable invention of the human race only an improved muck-rake? Is this the ground on which Orientals and Occidentals meet? Did God direct us so to get our living digging where we never planted,—and He would, perchance, reward us with lumps of gold?

God gave the righteous man a certificate entitling him to food and raiment, but the unrighteous man found a facsimile of the same in God's coffers, and appropriated it, and obtained food and raiment like the former. It is one of the most extensive systems of counterfeiting that the world has seen. I did not know that mankind were suffering for want of gold. I have seen a little of it. I know that it is very malleable, but not so malleable as wit. A grain of gold will gild a great surface, but not so much as a grain of wisdom.

The gold-digger in the ravines of the mountains is as much a gambler as his fellow in the saloons of San Francisco. What differences does it make whether you shake dirt or shake dice? If you win, society is the loser. The gold-digger is the enemy of the honest laborer, whatever checks and compensations there may be. It is not enough to tell me that you worked hard to get your gold. So does the Devil work hard. The way of transgressors may be hard in many respects. The humblest observer who goes to the mines sees and says that gold-digging is of the character of a lottery; the gold thus obtained is not the same thing with the wages of honest toil. But, practically, he forgets what he has seen, for he has seen only the fact, not the principle, and goes into trade there, that is, buys a ticket in what commonly proves another lottery, where the fact is not so obvious.

After reading Howitt's account of the Australian gold-diggings one evening, I had in my mind's eye, all night, the numerous valleys, with their streams, all cut up with foul pits, from ten to one hundred feet deep, and half a dozen feet across, as close as they can be dug, and partly filled with water,—the locality to which men furiously rush to probe for their fortunes,—uncertain where they shall break ground,—not knowing but the gold is under their camp itself,—sometimes digging one hundred and sixty feet before they strike the vein, or then missing it by a foot,—turned into demons, and regardless of each others' rights, in their thirst for riches, —whole valleys, for thirty miles, suddenly honeycombed by the pits of the miners, so that even hundreds are drowned in them,—standing in water, and covered with mud and clay, they work night and day, dying of exposure and disease. Having read this, and partly forgotten it, I was thinking, accidentally, of my own unsatisfactory life, doing as others do; and with that vision of the digging still before me, I asked myself why I might not be washing some gold daily, though it were only the finest particles,—why I might not sink a shaft down to the gold within me, and work that mine. *There* is a Ballarat, a Bendigo for you,—what though it were a sulky-gully? At any rate, I might pursue some path, however solitary and narrow and crooked, in which I could walk with love and reverence. Wherever a man separates from the multitude, and goes his own way in this mood, there indeed is a fork in the road, though ordinary travelers may see only a gap in the paling. His solitary path across-lots will turn out the *higher way* of the two.

Men rush to California and Australia as if the true gold were to be found in that direction; but that is to go to the very opposite extreme to where it lies. They go prospecting farther and farther away from the true lead, and are most unfortunate when they think themselves most successful. Is not our *native* soil auriferous? Does not a stream from the golden mountains flow through our native valley? and has not this for more than geologic ages been bringing down the shining particles and forming the nuggets for us? Yet, strange to tell, if a digger steal away, prospecting for this true gold, into the unexplored solitudes around us, there is no danger that any will dog his steps, and endeavor to supplant him. He may claim and undermine the whole valley even, both the cultivated and the uncultivated portions, his whole life long in peace, for no one will ever dispute his claim. They will not mind his cradles or his toms. He is not confined to a claim twelve feet square, as at Ballarat, but may mine anywhere, and wash the whole wide world in his tom.

Howitt says of the man who found the great nugget which weighed twenty-eight pounds, at the Bendigo diggings in Australia: "He soon began to drink; got a horse, and rode all about, generally at full gallop, and, when he met people, called out to inquire if they knew who he was, and then kindly informed them that he was 'the bloody wretch that had found the nugget.' At last he rode full speed against a tree, and nearly knocked his brains out." I think, however, there was no danger of that, for he had already knocked his brains out against the nugget. Howitt adds, "He is a hopelessly ruined man." But he is a type of the class. They are all fast men. Hear some of the names of the places where they dig: "Jackass Flat,"—"Sheep's-Head Gully,"—"Murderer's Bar," etc. Is there no satire in these names? Let them carry their ill-gotten wealth where they will, I am thinking it will still be "Jackass Flat," if not "Murderer's Bar," where they live.

The last resource of our energy has been the robbing of graveyards on the Isthmus of Darien, an enterprise which appears to be but in its infancy; for, according to late accounts, an act has passed its second
reading in the legislature of New Granada, regulating
this kind of mining; and a correspondent of the *Tribune*
writes: "In the dry season, when the weather will permit
of the country being properly prospected, no doubt
other rich *guacas* [that is, graveyards] will be found." To
emigrants he says: "Do not come before December; take
the Isthmus route in preference to the Boca del Toro
one; bring no useless baggage, and do not cumber yourself with a tent; but a good pair of blankets will be necessary; a pick, shovel, and axe of good material will be
almost all that is required:" advice which might have
been taken from the "Burker's Guide." And he con-
cludes with this line in Italics and small capitals: "*If you
are doing well at home,* STAY THERE," which may fairly be
interpreted to mean, "If you are getting a good living by
robbing graveyards at home, stay there."

But why go to California for a text? She is the child
of New England, bred at her own school and church.

It is remarkable that among all the preachers there
are so few moral teachers. The prophets are employed in
excusing the ways of men. Most reverend seniors, the
illuminati of the age, tell me, with a gracious, reminiscent
smile, betwixt an aspiration and a shudder, not to be too
tender about these things,—to lump all that, that is,
make a lump of gold of it. The highest advice I have
heard on these subjects was groveling. The burden of it

was,—It is not worth your while to undertake to reform the world in this particular. Do not ask how your bread is buttered; it will make you sick, if you do—and the like. A man had better starve at once than lose his innocence in the process of getting his bread. If within the sophisticated man there is not an unsophisticated one, then he is but one of the Devil's angels. As we grow old, we live more coarsely, we relax a little in our disciplines, and, to some extent, cease to obey our finest instincts. But we should be fastidious to the extreme of sanity, disregarding the gibes of those who are more unfortunate than ourselves.

In our science and philosophy, even, there is commonly no true and absolute account of things. The spirit of sect and bigotry has planted its hoof amid the stars. You have only to discuss the problem, whether the stars are inhabited or not, in order to discover it. Why must we daub the heavens as well as the earth? It was an unfortunate discovery that Dr. Kane was a Mason, and that Sir John Franklin was another. But it was a more cruel suggestion that possibly that was the reason why the former went in search of the latter. There is not a popular magazine in this country that would dare to print a child's thought on important subjects without comment. It must be submitted to the D. D.'s. I would it were the chicka-dee-dees.

You come from attending the funeral of mankind to attend to a natural phenomenon. A little thought is sexton to all the world.

I hardly know an *intellectual* man, even, who is so

broad and truly liberal that you can think aloud in his society. Most with whom you endeavor to talk soon come to a stand against some institution in which they appear to hold stock,—that is, some particular, not universal, way of viewing things. They will continually thrust their own low roof, with its narrow skylight, between you and the sky, when it is the unobstructed heavens you would view. Get out of the way with your cobwebs, wash your windows, I say! In some lyceums they tell me that they have voted to exclude the subject of religion. But how do I know what their religion is, and when I am near to or far from it? I have walked into such an arena and done my best to make a clean breast of what religion I have experienced, and the audience never suspected what I was about. The lecture was as harmless as moonshine to them. Whereas, if I had read to them the biography of the greatest scamps in history, they might have thought that I had written the lives of the deacons of their church. Ordinarily, the inquiry is, Where did you come from? or, Where are you going? That was a more pertinent question which I overheard one of my auditors put to another once,—"What does he lecture for?" It made me quake in my shoes.

To speak impartially, the best men that I know are not serene, a world in themselves. For the most part, they dwell in forms, and flatter and study effect only more finely than the rest. We select granite for the underpinning of our houses and barns; we build fences of stone; but we do not ourselves rest on an underpinning of granitic truth, the lowest primitive rock. Our sills are rotten. What stuff is the man made of who is not coexistent in our thought with the purest and subtilest truth? I often accuse my finest acquaintances of an immense frivolity; for, while there are manners and compliments we do not meet, we do not teach one another the lessons of honesty and sincerity that the brutes do, or of steadiness and solidity that the rocks do. The fault is commonly mutual, however; for we do not habitually demand any more of each other.

That excitement about Kossuth, consider how characteristic, but superficial, it was!—only another kind of politics or dancing. Men were making speeches to him all over the country, but each expressed only the thought, or the want of thought, of the multitude. No man stood on truth. They were merely banded together, as usual one leaning on another, and all together on nothing; as the Hindoos made the world rest on an elephant, the elephant on a tortoise, and the tortoise on a serpent, and had nothing to put under the serpent. For all fruit of that stir we have the Kossuth hat.

Just so hollow and ineffectual, for the most part, is our ordinary conversation. Surface meets surface. When our life ceases to be inward and private, conversation degenerates into mere gossip. We rarely meet a man who can tell us any news which he has not read in a newspaper, or been told by his neighbor; and, for the most part, the only difference between us and our fellow is that he has seen the newspaper, or been out to tea, and we have not. In proportion as our inward life fails, we go more constantly and desperately to the post-office. You may depend on it, that the poor fellow who walks away with the greatest number of letters proud of his extensive correspondence has not heard from himself this long while.

I do not know but it is too much to read one newspaper a week. I have tried it recently, and for so long it seems to me that I have not dwelt in my native region. The sun, the clouds, the snow, the trees say not so much to me. You cannot serve two masters. It requires more than a day's devotion to know and to possess the wealth of a day.

We may well be ashamed to tell what things we have read or heard in our day. I do not know why my news should be so trivial,—considering what one's dreams and expectations are, why the developments should be so paltry. The news we hear, for the most part, is not news to our genius. It is the stalest repetition. You are often tempted to ask why such stress is laid on a particular experience which you have had,—that, after twenty-five years, you should meet Hobbins, Registrar of Deeds, again on the sidewalk. Have you not budged an inch, then? Such is the daily news. Its facts appear to float in the atmosphere, insignificant as the sporules of fungi, and impinge on some neglected *thallus*, or surface of our minds, which affords a basis for them, and hence a parasitic growth. We should wash ourselves clean of such news. Of what consequence, though our planet explode, if there is no character involved in the explosion? In health we have not the least curiosity about such events. We do not live for idle amusement. I would not run round a corner to see the world blow up.

All summer, and far into the autumn, perchance, you unconsciously went by the newspapers and the news, and now you find it was because the morning and the evening were full of news to you. Your walks were full of incidents. You attended, not to the affairs of Europe, but to your own affairs in Massachusetts fields. If you chance to live and move and have your being in that thin stratum in which the events that make the news transpire,—thinner than the paper on which it is printed,—then these things will fill the world for you; but if you soar about or dive below that plane, you cannot remember nor be reminded of them. Really to see the sun rise or go down every day, so to relate ourselves to a universal fact, would preserve us sane forever. Nations! What are nations? Tartars, and Huns, and Chinamen! Like insects, they swarm. The historian strives in vain to make them memorable. It is for want of a man that there are so many men. It is individuals that populate the world. Any man thinking may say with the Spirit of Lodin,—

> "I look down from my height on nations,
> And they become ashes before me;—
> Calm is my dwelling in the clouds;
> Pleasant are the great fields of my rest."

Pray, let us live without being drawn by dogs, Esquimaux-fashion, tearing over hill and dale, and biting each other's ears.

Not without a slight shudder at the danger, I often

perceive how near I had come to admitting into my
mind the details of some trivial affair,—the news of the
street; and I am astonished to observe how willing men
are to lumber their minds with such rubbish,—to
permit idle rumors and incidents of the most insignificant kind to intrude on ground which should be sacred
to thought. Shall the mind be a public arena, where the
affairs of the street and the gossip of the tea-table
chiefly are discussed? Or shall it be a quarter of heaven
itself,—an hypæthral temple, consecrated to the service
of the gods? I find it so difficult to dispose of the few
facts which to me are significant, that I hesitate to
burden my attention with those which are insignificant,
which only a divine mind could illustrate. Such is, for
the most part, the news in newspapers and conversation.
It is important to preserve the mind's chastity in this respect. Think of admitting the details of a single case of
the criminal court into our thoughts, to stalk profanely
through their very *sanctum sanctorum* for an hour, ay, for
many hours! to make a very bar-room of the mind's in-
most apartment, as if for so long the dust of the street
had occupied us,—the very street itself, with all its
travel, its bustle, and filth, had passed through our
thoughts' shrine! Would it not be an intellectual and
moral suicide? When I have been compelled to sit spectator and auditor in a court room for some hours, and
have seen my neighbors, who were not compelled,
stealing in from time to time, and tiptoeing about with
washed hands and faces, it has appeared to my mind's
eye, that, when they took off their hats, their ears sud-

denly expanded into vast hoppers for sound, between which even their narrow heads were crowded. Like the vanes of windmills, they caught the broad but shallow stream of sound, which, after a few titillating gyrations in their coggy brains, passed out the other side. I wondered if, when they got home, they were as careful to wash their ears as before their hands and faces. It has seemed to me, at such a time, that the auditors and the witnesses, the jury and the counsel, the judge and the criminal at the bar,—if I may presume him guilty before he is convicted,—were all equally criminal, and a thunderbolt might be expected to descend and consume them all together.

By all kinds of traps and signboards, threatening the extreme penalty of the divine law, exclude such trespassers from the only ground which can be sacred to you. It is so hard to forget what it is worse than useless to remember! If I am to be a thoroughfare, I prefer that it be of the mountain-brooks, the Parnassian streams, and not the town-sewers. There is inspiration, that gossip which comes to the ear of the attentive mind from the courts of heaven. There is the profane and stale revelation of the bar-room and the police court. The same ear is fitted to receive both communications. Only the character of the hearer determines to which it shall be open, and to which closed. I believe that the mind can be permanently profaned by the habit of attending to trivial things, so that all our thoughts shall be tinged with triviality. Our very intellect shall be macadamized, as it were,—its foundation broken into fragments for the wheels of travel to roll over; and if you would know what will make the most durable pavement, surpassing rolled stones, spruce blocks, and asphaltum, you have only to look into some of our minds which have been subjected to this treatment so long.

If we have thus desecrated ourselves,—as who has not?—the remedy will be wariness and devotion to re-consecrate ourselves, and make once more a fane of the mind. We should treat our minds, that is, ourselves, as in-nocent and ingenuous children, whose guardians we are, and be careful what objects and what subjects we thrust on their attention. Read not the Times. Read the Eter-nities. Conventionalities are at length as bad as impuri-ties. Even the facts of science may dust the mind by their dryness, unless they are in a sense effaced each morning, or rather rendered fertile by the dews of fresh and living truth. Knowledge does not come to us by de-tails, but in flashes of light from heaven. Yes, every thought that passes through the mind helps to wear and tear it, and to deepen the ruts, which, as in the streets of Pompeii, evince how much it has been used. How many things there are concerning which we might well delib-erate whether we had better know them,—had better let their peddling-carts be driven, even at the slowest trot or walk, over that bridge of glorious span by which we trust to pass at last from the farthest brink of time to the nearest shore of eternity! Have we no culture, no re-finement,—but skill only to live coarsely and serve the Devil?—to acquire a little worldly wealth, or fame, or liberty, and make a false show with it, as if we were all husk and shell, with no tender and living kernel to us? Shall our institutions be like those chestnut-burs which contain abortive nuts, perfect only to prick the fingers?

America is said to be the arena on which the battle of freedom is to be fought; but surely it cannot be freedom in a merely political sense that is meant. Even if we grant that the American has freed himself from a political tyrant, he is still the slave of an economical and moral tyrant. Now that the republic—the *res publica*—has been settled, it is time to look after *res privata*,—the private state,—to see, as the Roman senate charged its consuls, "*ne quid res privata detrimenti caperet,*" that the *private* state receive no detriment.

Do we call this the land of the free? What is it to be free from King George and continue the slaves of King Prejudice? What is it to be born free and not live free? What is the value of any political freedom, but as a means to moral freedom? Is it a freedom to be slaves, or a freedom to be free, of which we boast? We are a nation of politicians, concerned about the outmost defenses only of freedom. It is our children's children who may perchance be really free. We tax ourselves unjustly. There is a part of us which is not represented. It is taxation without representation. We quarter troops, we quarter fools and cattle of all sorts upon ourselves. We quarter our gross bodies on our poor souls, till the former eat up all the latter's substance.

With respect to a true culture and manhood, we are essentially provincial still, not metropolitan,—mere Jonathans. We are provincial, because we do not find at home our standards; because we do not worship truth, but the reflection of truth; because we are warped and narrowed by an exclusive devotion to trade and commerce and manufactures and agriculture and the like, which are but means, and not the end.

So is the English Parliament provincial. Mere country-bumpkins, they betray themselves, when any more important question arises for them to settle, the Irish question, for instance,—the English question why did I not say? Their natures are subdued to what they work in. Their "good breeding" respects only secondary objects. The finest manners in the world are awkwardness and fatuity when contrasted with a finer intelligence. They appear but as the fashions of past days,—mere courtliness, knee-buckles and small-clothes, out of date. It is the vice, but not the excellence of manners, that they are continually being deserted by the character; they are cast-off clothes or shells, claiming the respect which belonged to the living creature. You are presented with the shell instead of the meat, and it is no excuse generally, that, in the case of some fishes, the shells are of more worth than the meat. The man who thrusts his manners upon me does as if he were to insist on introducing me to his cabinet of curiosities, when I wished to see himself. It was not in this sense that the poet Decker called Christ "the first true gentleman that ever breathed." I repeat that in this sense the most splendid court in Christendom is provincial, having authority to consult about Transalpine interests only, and not the affairs of Rome. A praetor or proconsul would suffice to settle the questions which absorb the attention of the English Parliament and the American Congress.

Government and legislation: these I thought were respectable professions. We have heard of heaven-born Numas, Lycurguses, and Solons, in the history of the world, whose *names* at least may stand for ideal legislators; but think of legislating to *regulate* the breeding of slaves, or the exportation of tobacco! What have divine legislators to do with the exportation or the importation of tobacco? what humane ones with the breeding of slaves? Suppose you were to submit the question to any son of God,—and has He no children in the nineteenth century? is it a family which is extinct?—in what condition would you get it again? What shall a State like Virginia say for itself at the last day, in which these have been the principal, the staple productions? What ground is there for patriotism in such a State? I derive the facts from statistical tables which the States themselves have published.

A commerce that whitens every sea in quest of nuts and raisins, and makes slaves of its sailors for this purpose! I saw, the other day, a vessel which had been wrecked, and many lives lost, and her cargo of rags, juniper-berries, and bitter almonds were strewn along the shore. It seemed hardly worth the while to tempt the dangers of the sea between Leghorn and New York for the sake of a cargo of juniper-berries and bitter almonds. America sending to the Old World for her bitters! Is not the sea-brine, is not shipwreck, bitter enough to make the cup of life go down here? Yet such, to a great extent, is our boasted commerce; and there are those who style themselves statesmen and philosophers who are so blind as to think that progress and civilization depend on precisely this kind of interchange and activity,—the activity of flies about a molasses-hoghead. Very well, observes one, if men were oysters. And very well, answer I, if men were mosquitoes.

Lieutenant Herndon, whom our Government sent to explore the Amazon, and, it is said, to extend the area of slavery, observed that there was wanting there "an industrious and active population, who know what the comforts of life are, and who have artificial wants to draw out the great resources of the country." But what are the "artificial wants" to be encouraged? Not the love of luxuries, like the tobacco and slaves of, I believe, his native Virginia, nor the ice and granite and other material wealth of our native New England; nor are "the great resources of a country" that fertility or barrenness of soil which produces these. The chief want, in every State that I have been into, was a high and earnest purpose in its inhabitants. This alone draws out "the great resources" of Nature, and at last taxes her beyond her resources; for man naturally dies out of her. When we want sugar-plums, then the great resources of a world are taxed and drawn out, and the result, or staple production, is, not slaves, nor operatives, but men,—those rare fruits called heroes, saints, poets, philosophers, and redeemers.

In short, as a snow-drift is formed where there is a lull in the wind, so, one would say, where there is a lull of truth, an institution springs up. But the truth blows right on over it, nevertheless, and at length blows it down.

What is called politics is comparatively something so superficial and inhuman, that practically I have never fairly recognized that it concerns me at all. The newspapers, I perceive, devote some of their columns specially to politics or government without charge; and this, one would say, is all that saves it; but as I love literature and to some extent the truth also, I never read those columns at any rate. I do not wish to blunt my sense of right so much. I have not got to answer for having read a single President's Message. A strange age of the world this, when empires, kingdoms, and republics come a-begging to a private man's door, and utter their complaints at his elbow! I cannot take up a newspaper but I find that some wretched government or other, hard pushed, and on its last legs, is interceding with me, the reader, to vote for it,—more importunate than an Italian beggar; and if I have a mind to look at its certificate, made, perchance, by some benevolent merchant's clerk, or the skipper that brought it over, for it cannot speak a word of English itself, I shall probably read of the eruption of some Vesuvius, or the overflowing of some Po, true or forged, which brought it into this condition. I do not hesitate, in such a case, to suggest work or the almshouse; or why not keep its castle in silence, as I do commonly? The poor President, what with preserving his popularity and doing his duty, is completely bewildered. The newspapers are the ruling power. Any other government is reduced to a few marines at Fort Independence. If a man neglects to read the *Daily Times,* government will go down on its knees to him, for this is the only treason in these days.

Those things which now most engage the attention of men, as politics and the daily routine, are, it is true, vital functions of human society, but should be unconsciously performed, like the corresponding functions of the physical body. They are *infra*-human, a kind of vegetation. I sometimes awake to a half-consciousness of them going on about me, as a man may become conscious of some of the processes of digestion in a morbid state, and so have the dyspepsia, as it is called. It is as if a thinker submitted himself to be rasped by the great gizzard of creation. Politics is, as it were, the gizzard of society, full of grit and gravel, and the two political parties are its two opposite halves,—sometimes split into quarters, it may be, which grind on each other. Not only individuals, but states, have thus a confirmed dyspepsia, which expresses itself, you can imagine by what sort of eloquence. Thus our life is not altogether a forgetting, but also, alas! to a great extent, a remembering, of that which we should never have been conscious of, certainly not in our waking hours. Why should we not meet, not always as dyspeptics, to tell our bad dreams, but sometimes as *eu*peptics, to congratulate each other on the ever-glorious morning? I do not make an exorbitant demand, surely.